ACUPUNCTURE FOR NEW PRACTITIONERS

of related interest

Needling Techniques for Acupuncturists
Basic Principles and Techniques
Editor in Chief: Professor Chang Xiaorong
ISBN 978 1 84819 057 3
eISBN 978 0 85701 045 2

Meridians and Acupoints
Edited by Zhu Bing and Wang Hongcai
Advisor: Cheng Xinnong
ISBN 978 1 84819 037 5
eISBN 978 0 85701 021 6

Acupuncture Therapeutics
Edited by Zhu Bing and Wang Hongcai
Advisor: Cheng Xinnong
ISBN 978 1 84819 039 9
eISBN 978 0 85701 018 6

I Ching Acupuncture – The Balance Method
Clinical Applications of the Ba Gua and I Ching
David Twicken
ISBN 978 1 84819 074 0
eISBN 978 0 85701 064 3

Relating to Clients
The Therapeutic Relationship for Complementary Therapists
Su Fox
ISBN 978 1 84310 615 9
eISBN 978 1 84642 718 3

'This is a thoughtful, practical and inspirational guide addressing many of the common issues that arise in the first years of practice. Using questions to help focus the reader and meaningful anecdotes to illustrate the journey to be travelled, John develops a blueprint for holistic development. It is a delight to read and will aid the path to artistry and mastery in one's professional role. How I wish it had been available to me in my early days of practice!'

– *Alison Gould, acupuncturist and Accreditation Officer for the British Acupuncture Accreditation Board*

'*Acupuncture for New Practitioners* is an acupuncture book like no other. It addresses intangible qualities that cannot be measured by test scores. Rather than tell us what to think or what to do, this wonderfully honest book by a wise and experienced practitioner instructs us on how to think and, perhaps more importantly, how to be. Every chapter contains pearls of wisdom, gently yet firmly guiding us toward finding our own truth, both as practitioners and as human beings. The author reminds us to be present in every moment and dares us to continue to learn and grow. He provides a pathway for fostering compassion, competence and confidence, and for transforming knowledge and skill into wisdom. This book will prove invaluable not only for new practitioners but also for those of us with decades of experience.'

– *Eugene London, DAOM, Dipl.Ac. (NCCAOM), L.Ac.*

ACUPUNCTURE FOR NEW PRACTITIONERS

John Hamwee

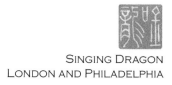

SINGING DRAGON
LONDON AND PHILADELPHIA

First published in 2012
by Singing Dragon
an imprint of Jessica Kingsley Publishers
116 Pentonville Road
London N1 9JB, UK
and
400 Market Street, Suite 400
Philadelphia, PA 19106, USA

www.singingdragon.com

Copyright © John Hamwee 2012

Library of Congress Cataloging in Publication Data
A CIP catalog record for this book is available from the Library of Congress

British Library Cataloguing in Publication Data
A CIP catalogue record for this book is available from the British Library

ISBN 978 1 84819 102 0
eISBN 978 0 85701 083 4

Printed and bound in Great Britain

Dedicated to

Aye Thandar Soe
Moe Moe Khin

and their colleagues at the
Watchet Jivitadana Sangha Hospital

CONTENTS

ACKNOWLEDGEMENTS

I learned almost everything I know about being a practitioner from Meriel Darby. Fritz Smith showed me the reality of energy in the human body, and demonstrated how to work with it. After I had been in practice some years, John and Angie Hicks finally taught me acupuncture. All of them gave freely of their wisdom and I hope I have managed to pass on some of it.

My teaching in Burma (Myanmar) would not be possible without the help and support of Sayadaw U. Lakkhana, Dr U. Win Ko and Vispassana Hawaii, and I am very grateful to them.

Jessica Kingsley received the book in a way that authors dream of but rarely experience.

PREFACE

There is a moment when you bend over a point, needle in hand, which takes a certain amount of courage. You are about to take decisive action, backing your judgement, realising that if you are wrong it will be your patient who will suffer the consequences. For just as you know that the treatment can really help a person get better, so you are bound to acknowledge that it can also make her worse. Then, perhaps with a slight pause as if in deference to this responsibility, you go ahead and insert the needle. And you do it many times during a working day. It is demanding work.

I know what it takes to be able to do this, day in day out. I qualified as an acupuncturist in my mid forties and by then I had already had two jobs in which I managed big projects and dealt with large sums of money. But even now, 20 years later, I look back on the decisions I took then as easier and less weighty than those I now take every day in the treatment room. For although I sometimes used to worry about those decisions, it was as nothing compared to the concern I feel when I'm not at all sure that I've done a good treatment and I know my patient will have to live with it, having to cope with the strains of his or her own life with the added handicap of an energy system unbalanced by my treatment. And in most cases my patient will already be struggling with some condition which made life difficult enough as it was.

What I have learned, after many years of trial and error, is how to manage this responsibility; how to make the work less stressful, more satisfying, and thereby more effective too.

This book does not give you new information about acupuncture; if you've qualified, or are in the late stages of training, you know enough of the theory and techniques to be safe and competent. It is about how to practise; how to work each day in a way that nourishes you and improves your treatments. It comes from my reflections on having walked the path before you and finding it often hard, always rewarding, but never less than challenging.

This book was born on a plane flying high over the Bay of Bengal. I was on my way home from Myanmar, formerly known as Burma, where I had been working for two weeks with four other Western acupuncturists. We treated first in a hospital on the banks of the Irrawaddy river, and then in a monastery in a small village. It was a moving and life-changing experience.

The patients came in waves. I was used to treating no more than nine people in a day; in Myanmar I treated 26 on the first day and the number rose from then on. I was used to treating a limited range of conditions; there, I saw babies with enormous tumours, women who had given birth to 12 children, and monks with crippled knees. I was used to working on my own in the treatment room; there, I was crowded in with maybe 50 people, patients and practitioners, and there were faces peering in through every window. And another key difference was that I was used to teaching students; there, I had to teach young practitioners. For we were accompanied at work by two, three, or more young acupuncturists who were acting as our assistants, helping with translation and observing what we were doing.

I hadn't known I was going to have to do that but there I was, having to treat enormous numbers of people quickly without being able to speak their language, while teaching practitioners at the same time. Well, I just did it. There was no choice. There were the patients and there were the acupuncturists watching, and the long day stretched out ahead. I didn't have time to think; I just said and did what instinctively seemed appropriate at the time and hoped that the students were learning something useful.

On the plane back home I did have time to think, so I cast my mind back over the hectic, exhausting, exhilarating time I had just had and thought to myself, 'What did I teach them, exactly?' As I mulled over the question I realised that some patterns had emerged. There were ideas, concepts, ways of thinking about a patient, of testing a diagnosis, of evaluating a treatment, which I had repeated over and over again as different students joined me on different days. And the whole experience led me to realise that these students were at a particular and interesting stage of their training. They knew what they had learned at college, and knew it well. Equally obviously, they could not know what can't be taught at college because it depends on having some experience of practice.

It slowly dawned on me that there is a natural syllabus, so to speak, for acupuncturists in the first few years of their careers; that there are things they need to learn which can't be taught sooner, and which they will not need to be taught later, because when they have been working for some years they will have discovered them for themselves. That therefore it would be useful to novice practitioners to set these things out, so that they could learn the lessons of practice perhaps a little more quickly and a little more fully than they could on their own. And I hoped it might save them some of the difficulties and anxieties of finding all these things out for themselves through trial and sometimes painful error.

I wrote it originally for the young acupuncturists in Myanmar, mainly as a kind of thank-you for all the warmth and kindness they extended to me, for which I will always be in their debt. But I send it out now to a wider audience, hoping that it will make your early years of practice less stressful, more enjoyable, and better for your own health as well as for that of your patients.

CHAPTER 1

IN THE MOMENT

A pretty good test of how well you are working, I have found, is how you feel at the end of a day. If you've been unsure about what you've done, concerned that some of your patients aren't doing as well as you (or they) hoped, if you are not confident in your diagnoses, and have the feeling that you haven't quite got to the bottom of what's going on, then the chances are that you'll be weary and even a little dispirited as you close the door of your treatment room. By contrast, the best practitioner I ever observed, when I was in my last year as a student, was in his late sixties. He treated 14 people straight off, each one a crafted, individualised treatment – I was exhausted just watching – and there was a bounce in his walk as he left his clinic at the end of the day. This book is about how to finish a full day's work like him, feeling better than when you started.

You may regard this as an idealistic aspiration or a needless luxury. It may be so for other jobs, but for we acupuncturists is nothing of the sort; in fact, it is essential.

For we work with energy. It is what we do. It is all we do. It is how we stimulate healing of all kinds. If we cannot manage our own energy then our patients may reasonably question whether we can manage theirs. Would you invest your money with a financial advisor who has trouble paying his household bills? Or trust the advice of a director of human resources who can't get on with his own staff? There is an irreducible principle here.

There is a well-known story about Mahatma Gandhi. Local people used to come to him and ask him for all kinds of help and advice. One day a mother brought her five-year-old child. 'Mahatma,' she said, 'will you please tell my son to stop eating sugar? I tell him it is very bad for him but he won't listen to me. I am sure he will listen to you.'

There was a silence which lasted longer than she expected. Then Gandhi said, 'Come back next week,' and waved the woman away.

She returned as she'd been told and Gandhi bent down to the child and said, 'Now listen to me. You must not eat sugar. Your mother and I agree it is very bad for you, so you must do as we say,' and he looked the boy deep into his eyes to make sure he took it seriously.

The mother thanked him, and as she turned to go she said, 'Mahatma, may I ask why you made me come back, why you didn't say that to my son last week?'

'Oh,' he replied. 'Last week I had not given up eating sugar.'

As Americans say, you have to walk the talk. But what is the talk, exactly? To answer that question we need to take full account of the most basic principles of acupuncture. For this system of medicine to work at all, as we know it does, a human being must have an energy body as well as a physical body. That is, just as we have bones and muscles, tendons and ligaments, organs and nerves, which are systematically connected, so too we have flows of energy which are organised in coherent and predictable ways. These flows animate the structure; without them it is merely inert matter. And when the flows become disturbed or disorganised in some way, the effect is a diminution in our ability to function well in the world. We become vulnerable to pathogens, we fall ill, mentally or physically, we lose the full range of our functions, again either physically or mentally, and in the long term there may well be irreversible tissue change. Valerie V. Hunt was a professor of physiology at three prestigious American universities; she wrote, 'Probably illness is a disturbance first in the energy field and healing is a restoration of that field to health…when tissue is diseased, the problem is already far advanced' (Hunt 1989, p.244).

In other words, what we are doing is restoring the patient's energy body (what Professor Hunt calls the 'energy field') to as near its naturally organised state as possible. This simple statement has some very important implications.

The first stems from the fact that we work in a room with a patient, normally alone together, for anything between 20 minutes and an hour.

In one of her well-known experiments, Professor Hunt put two people who did not know each other in a room, sitting back to back on two chairs. They did not talk or otherwise communicate. Both of them had electrodes attached all over them so that she could monitor changes in their energy bodies. What she observed was fascinating.

Occasionally, but rarely, there was no change in the energy bodies of either person. They simply didn't have any effect on each other. Most often, however, what happened is that both of their energy bodies changed, and however different they were at the start they ended up in a pretty similar state. It's as if the two people merged their energy bodies to reach a common, shared one; a bit like mixing blue and yellow paint and getting green. Finally, sometimes, the energy body of only one of the people changed, and it changed to become like the energy body of the other. In this case, it was as if the energy body of one person was so much stronger that it dominated the other, and took it over.

I am sure you recognise all this because we have all had these experiences ourselves, and not only in the treatment room. There are some people who, as we say, leave us cold. I imagine that this is one way of reporting that the two energy bodies have had no effect on each other. Then there are people with whom we feel better, bigger, more rounded, more relaxed, more at ease than when we are alone; I take this to be the feeling of having merged our energy body with that of another, as happens most powerfully and dramatically when we fall in love. It is a kind of intimacy that can happen even without touch. As it is somewhat mysterious to us we often use a metaphor to explain it, and call it 'chemistry'; perhaps to see it as a change in our energy bodies is no metaphor but a literal description of what has happened.

Then, finally, there are some people whose presence seems to overwhelm us in some way, normally making us feel uncomfortable. I'm thinking, for example, of people who always seem to stand a bit too close or those who make us tense or agitated even when we can't pinpoint anything they've said or done to make us feel this way. It often seems as if there is some vague lurking threat somewhere in the background. Maybe what we are noticing here is the sensation of having our energy body invaded by that of another, and one which is uncongenial at that.

Back to the treatment room. You may be thinking, 'I didn't realise my patient could be having such an effect on me.' Indeed, and I have more to say about that in a moment. But don't overlook the other side of the coin – the effect you may be having on your patient. If your energy body is disorganised, disturbed, distorted, then, according to Professor Hunt, you may be altering your patient's energy away from health and towards illness simply by your presence in the room for a substantial period of time. A serious issue, bearing in mind the most fundamental principle of the practice of medicine, 'do no harm'.

I said earlier that it is no trivial matter that your work should make you feel well and energised. That's because it is a sign that your own energy body is organised and strong, and so you can be sure that you have done no harm to your patients by your very presence. On the contrary, it has probably helped them to get better.

So your energy body needs to be in good shape for your day's work. Perhaps you are one of those lucky people who doesn't have to do anything to make it so; it is normally and naturally well. But for most of us it needs some attention. Just as we brush our teeth every day, we may need to have some daily practice which refreshes and revitalises the energy body – walking, meditating, doing taiji or qigong; and just as we also sometimes need to go to the dentist, so we need to have treatment ourselves every now and then if the energy body gets too far out of balance.

So far, so obvious; but I think there's more to it than that. I'm sure you have had the experience of a treatment that seemed somehow profound, where something happened which changed the atmosphere in the room, appeared to make it relax and soften, and the light became brighter too. It's hard to put into words actually. I can never predict when it is going to happen; it doesn't seem to have anything to do with the nature of the patient's complaint, or the nature of the patient either, if it comes to that. One of the most powerful instances in my practice was with a new patient, a middle-aged farm worker with a painful left hip and knee. She was not some new age devotee in the middle of a psycho-spiritual crisis, and as far as I could tell she had simply been working too hard at harvest time and needed rest, though that wasn't going to be possible for a few more weeks. So I did a very straightforward treatment, helping blood and Qi to flow through the joints. That's when it happened. A remarkable transformation took place. The strain in her face faded away and was replaced by a smile, her body seemed to lie more easily on the couch, her pulses improved beyond anything I had imagined or predicted, and then the whole room seemed to become more comfortable too.

And, of course, I was affected by it. She was the last patient at the end of a long day and before she arrived I was tired, slightly cross with myself that I had agreed to see her so late (at harvest time she couldn't come for treatment any earlier) and I was intent on getting through as quickly as possible and going home. By the time she left I felt wonderful, as if I had had a treatment myself. Which is probably not so far from the truth. For as her energy body became stronger, clearer and more powerful so it affected whatever was within range – which certainly included me and my energy body, and indeed the atmosphere in the room.

So that's how my teacher does it, I thought, as I locked up the clinic in the dusk; that's why he walks away from his work with a bounce in his step. His treatments are so powerful that he spends all day getting treated himself. It's a side effect, so to speak, of balancing the energy of others. As they get better, so does he.

Surely that's the way to do this work.

So what did I somehow manage to do with that farm worker which I clearly hadn't done with all my other patients that day? And how can you learn to do it yourself, and do it more often? And what can you do which will increase the chances of it happening every day? It will take the rest of this book to answer these questions fully, so for the rest of this introduction I want to talk about one fundamental issue which lies behind all the others in later chapters.

You may have heard the phrase, 'energy follows attention'. It took me years to work out what it means, but as it sums up much of what I want to say here I'll try to explain.

As a small experiment, put the fingertips of one hand on some kind of surface; the top of your knee (through clothing is fine), the cover of this book (that works better than a page), a table top or arm of your chair; anything within easy reach. Now concentrate on what you are feeling beneath your fingertips (you can move them about a bit if it helps). Is the surface smooth or rough? Warm or cold? Is it the same all over or are there differences? Is there some place which you find particularly attractive? Stop reading for a moment or two and take your eyes away from the page altogether, so you can really pay attention to the sensations.

Now, keeping you fingertips in the same place, I want you to think about how you use touch to locate points. Do you go straight to a point or do you slide your fingers along the skin until you find it? And if you slide, do you always feel along the skin in the same direction as the flow of energy in the meridian? Try to remember what you did last time you found Sp 6 or Pc 6 or Ki 7. Do you have some routine, feeling first proximal/distal and then anterior/ posterior, for example, or do you approach each point differently? Do you trust the anatomical location or do you need to feel the point under your fingertips before you place the needle there? Can you think of a recent example where you really felt a point and were absolutely sure that you knew where it was? What was that feeling, and what made you so sure?

These are all interesting questions but the point of the exercise was not to find answers to them but to get you thinking about something other than the sensation at your fingertips. I could have asked you to think about what you're going to cook tonight or how to phrase what you need to say in a letter you have to write (both familiar topics for me when I'm in the treatment room and I should be giving my full attention to my patient). Because, I feel safe in saying, while you were thinking of answers to these questions you stopped noticing the sensations under your fingertips. You can't do both at once, no one can. So if your mind is elsewhere when you are treating a patient you will miss the sensations under your fingers, and you need them in order to pick up vital information about his or her energy body – not just where the points are, but what the pulses reveal, the texture of the skin, the warmth of the flesh and a more general sense of excess or deficiency. If your attention is not with your patient but in your kitchen or at your desk then you simply miss the information you need in order to give an accurate and effective treatment.

Nor is it a matter of needing to pay attention only until you have reached your diagnosis. As you needle a point you need to know if that has changed the state of the patient's energy body. If there was no change then you haven't given the patient a treatment at all, and you'll need to know why. Did you simply miss the point, or was your diagnosis wrong in that it suggested a point which, in fact, made not the slightest difference to the state of your patient's energy body? And you'll only be able to answer that question if you were paying close attention as you needled, for only then will you know whether or not you hit the point.

And if there was a change, was it the change you expected? For example, you may have predicted that the pulse would rise and become fuller, and perhaps you also hoped that your patient's eyes would lose a certain dullness and gain a little sparkle. If this didn't happen, then again you need to reconsider; her energy body hasn't responded in quite the way you thought it would, so how can you change your approach to get the results you want? In short, you need to be constantly on the look-out for changes in the energy body, for they may come at any time. I'm sure you can think of instances from your own practice, but here are two recent ones from mine.

Not long ago a colleague was ill and off work for few weeks and she asked me to treat some of her patients while she was away. One of them was a nice, polite, middle-aged woman, softly spoken and very friendly towards me as we talked, saying how grateful she was that I had stepped in to help while her practitioner was not available, because she really needed regular treatment. She lay down on the couch, I took her pulses and looked at her tongue and I decided to start by needling a point with even technique. As I bent over her leg and touched the point with my finger I said, 'This first needle will be here; it'll stay in for a few minutes.' She reared up off the couch into a sitting position and practically shouted at me, 'Sally never does that!' The force of her energy hit me; it was almost like being slapped. I recoiled for a moment, shocked. And I knew immediately that my previous diagnosis was wrong. Up to that moment

I had not suspected that her energy body had such power, such pent-up pressure and strain, and that it desperately needed soothing and calming.

My other example is of a more subtle, more fleeting moment. A man in his late thirties, handsome, popular, successful, with two small children and a happy marriage. He comes for treatment because his skin occasionally erupts into the most violent red wheals which, when they were on his face, practically closed his eyes. He had been tested for all the usual allergies, but he had none, and there seemed to be no correlation between his skin complaint and times of stress. Not that he seemed to feel stress particularly; he appeared to be a warm, relaxed, happy-go-lucky kind of person.

Then, one day, when he'd just got back from his family holiday in France and he was telling me what a good time they'd all had, and how his skin had not been a problem at all, he looked away as he finished what he was saying and there flashed across his face an expression of such utter sadness, loneliness and hopelessness that I was stunned. I could hardly believe it; what I'd seen was so incongruous, so dissonant with what he'd been telling me and with the way I'd always regarded him. But it was unmistakable, and from then on I treated not the cheerful front man but the desperate one behind.

It is so easy to forget that energy moves fast. Blink, and you can miss it. Even when a patient is very depleted and one treatment can't make very much difference, still, if your point selection is accurate there will be a change, suddenly and unmistakably present in front of your eyes and under your fingers. It is in the very nature of energy medicine that it has this practically instantaneous effect – think of how the pulse responds so immediately to a needle. I am constantly amazed by it. So, as a practitioner of energy medicine you have to stay alert.

It sounds simple enough, but it isn't always easy. For one thing your attention is bound to drift off from time to time. You won't be able to help it. It happens to us all. But if you are alert you'll notice that you are suddenly thinking about your holiday, or what you forgot to say to someone yesterday, and you can bring your attention back again. And once you get into the habit you don't need to wait for your patient to wake you up by saying something which interrupts your reverie; you can catch it yourself within moments.

You might think that it sounds like hard work; that you'll have to concentrate the whole time and watch your patient like a hawk. It isn't like that at all. It's actually more a matter of learning to relax. Most of the time we all live with an endless stream of thoughts chattering through our heads, and we pay close attention to those thoughts, listening to them, evaluating them, taking them so seriously. It's practically a full-time job. The trick is to shift your attention from your thoughts to your sensations. Notice what you see when you look at your patient – ah, one shoulder is a lot higher than the other, almost as if one side of his body has crumpled up. Notice what you feel under your hands – ah, her skin is cold and clammy, even though it's a warm day. Notice what you hear in his voice, irrespective of what he is saying – ah, he's telling me about the time his wife and children were late home and he didn't know what had happened to them and he was concerned for their safety. But as he speaks he seems to be furious about it. Once you have really noticed, then it is usually pretty obvious what treatment you need to do; the observation itself brings a point or points to mind. Your knowledge and experience is working away in the background without any real effort on your part.

If, on the other hand, you haven't noticed anything, then the options are almost limitless, and you can spend enormous amounts of time and effort cudgelling your brain into choosing amongst them; and, ironically, the more you think about what treatment to do the less likely you are to pick up the messages which your patient's mind, body and spirit are sending you, and practically begging you to hear.

It really does take the effort out of working (well, much of it anyway). For, again, there is a kind of relaxation in simply responding to what your patient, involuntarily and unconsciously, is asking you to do. You can trust it in a way that you can't trust what they tell you. Not that your patients are deliberately trying to mislead you, but they often ignore what to you is crucial information or they conceal what they think you won't approve of. Sometimes their personalities distort what they are telling you; some put a brave face on things while others demand sympathy for any difficulty they encounter. All this gets in the way of you being able to see what they really need. It is so easy to get caught up in their stories and fail to notice the information which their energy bodies are communicating; information which bypasses endless theorising about what could be happening and what might be a good treatment. This kind of information avoids the doubt and worry which can linger long after you've taken the needles out. There is a kind of simple knowing about it.

Of course, like any new skill, it takes time and practice to acquire, and even though I've been working in this way for many years now, I know that I could do it a lot better than I do. But still, the sooner you start out on this road the further you'll travel.

And you may also be able to travel on it for longer. For after some years in practice there are practitioners who suffer from a kind of exhaustion, often called 'burn out'. They can no longer cope with the pressure of treating patients who are unwell and who depend on them to get better. As a result, they either stop working altogether or drastically cut the amount of work they do. Of course, being an acupuncturist is a demanding job, but there is something wrong if it is harmful to its practitioners. What is wrong, often, is that they are trying to work out what is the correct treatment for each individual patient, hour after hour, day after day, in the full knowledge that they might get it wrong and that the patient will fail to get better as a result. It's a very heavy burden to carry. If, by contrast, practitioners simply notice what the energy body is requesting, and respond to that request, then what is there to exhaust them? What they are doing, all they are doing, is as simple as passing a drink to someone who is thirsty.

Stay in the moment, that's all. Be aware of what is happening moment by moment in the treatment room. It sounds ridiculously simple. After all those years spent learning syndromes or stems and branches or constitutional factors it seems too simple. But those diagnostic methods you learned haven't been wasted; they are being used all the time to inform what it is you notice. I am only suggesting that you put them in the background rather than have them in the forefront of your mind. Try it. I think you'll find that work becomes easier and more powerful and that you'll feel much lighter about acupuncture, both in the treatment room and as a life's work.

Chapter 2

BEING YOURSELF

There's a lot going on in the first few years after qualification. You're building up a practice, worrying that your skills aren't good enough, finding out that not everything you were taught at college works all the time, and generally finding your way along a new and unfamiliar path – and pretty much in the dark, it sometimes seems.

In the early years you are bound to be deeply influenced by the training you received and by the practitioner who has treated you. Between them, they have shown you how to do it. You know perfectly well that there are other styles of acupuncture but you don't know much about them, certainly not enough to use them, and anyway you've seen such wonderful results from the kind of acupuncture you do know, why would you go chasing after something else?

So far, so sensible. But as you work you will find that you just can't get comfortable with some of the things you've been taught. My initial training was at a college which taught only one form of diagnosis – which was to decide whether the patient had a fundamental imbalance in one of five energies, Wood, Fire, Earth, Metal and

Water (sometimes called Five Element Constitutional Acupuncture or Leamington Acupuncture). That was all. The theory was that such a diagnosis was adequate, indeed essential, for any condition your patient brought to you: infertility, a bad back, tinnitus, migraines, irritable bowel, you name it. Provided the diagnosis was accurate, I was taught, treatment based on that diagnosis would work and the patient would get better.

I have colleagues who practise this style of acupuncture and I have great respect for them. I know they get good results, but I can't do it. For one thing, I just can't bring myself to believe that one kind of diagnosis fits all, that it works for everything and anything. For another, which I'm sure is not unconnected, I found I wasn't any good at it. That is, with the majority of my patients I couldn't tell which of the five energies or elements was fundamentally imbalanced (still can't, actually). For me, it's a bit like trying to do a crossword; even when I've seen the answers I still can't work out the clues. The last straw came when a colleague, expert in this kind of diagnosis, told me that she was sure that the key element of an old and close friend was Earth. I was astonished. I believed her, but I had never even suspected that to be the case. In fact, I could make what I considered was a more plausible case for any of the others! That was the end for me; I knew I could no longer go on trying to practise the kind of acupuncture I'd been taught.

I'm not suggesting that if you're finding what you've been trained to do difficult, and you're making mistakes, then you simply give up on it. But nor do you have to go through years of self-doubt, frustration, and even depression if, like me, you happen to have studied a form of acupuncture that doesn't really suit you. There are plenty more styles out there, and because you already know the points and their locations, the basic pulse qualities and so on, it's not that hard to learn them. What's more, provided you honour the basic principles and don't run counter to centuries of wisdom, randomly deciding, for example, that Sp 5 is better than Sp 10 for blood conditions, then it is absolutely alright to find your own way.

For example, if you were to find that you are not comfortable with diagnosis by syndromes you can still clear pathogens, decide if Yin or Yang is deficient or in excess, and treat the organ which seems to need help. That'll work. Or if you have trouble, as I did, with the idea of choosing one element to treat, then you can treat whichever ones seems to you weak or deficient. That'll work too. After all, if you take the theory at its most basic, energy flows through each element in turn, so it should get to where it's needed sooner or later.

The point I'm making is that you will get better results by practising in a way that makes sense to you and with which you are comfortable, than if you strain to do what you've been taught even though it doesn't suit you. And, when you think about it, there are so many different styles of acupuncture that it simply cannot be true that one of them works and the others don't; nor that they, and only they, constitute the full set of legitimate and effective ones. It is much more realistic to think that there are many, many ways of using needles and moxa to change a patient's energy body in the direction of health and healing, and that as long as you work in a way which is consistent with the core principles of this system of medicine, it is perfectly alright to find your own way of doing it.

Apart from anything else, this approach leads you to recognise your own limitations, and there is always wisdom in that. I remember working with one of my teachers and asking him why he'd chosen a particular point when I thought that there was an obvious alternative which would do the job better. 'You're quite right,' he said. 'But I always have trouble finding that point, so I do this one instead. It's better to hit the slightly less good point, I think, than to miss the better one.' Quite so.

All this is to urge you to use what you discover about your weaknesses, your limitations and your failures as a practitioner, not in order to create some kind of story about how you're not good enough, or you've never been a success, or how you should have listened to those who told you it was crazy to become an acupuncturist in the first place – whatever kind of story you usually tell yourself – but to use what you discover in order to choose a way of working that suits you, that builds on your strengths and avoids your limitations. Why not? There's no obvious merit in doing what you're not much good at while steering clear of what you are.

This issue affects everything. Let me take as one example the time you allocate for a treatment. The range I have seen personally is enormous, from 10 to 60 minutes. Why, for example, would you choose 60? Leaving aside that you might want to be sure to have a break between patients, the basic reason is to have a lot of time to talk. And why would you need that? Fundamentally, because you see your work in a very particular way, a way that can be characterised as follows.

You feel the need to get to know your patient quite intimately. You probably do not look for a standard diagnosis, and you are certainly open to having fresh ideas at each and every session. You may well have the conviction that, however straightforward the presenting complaint seems to be, it will have important psychological and maybe even spiritual dimensions, and that to ignore these would be to limit the power and potential of your treatment. In fact, when you reflect on your patients, you realise that for quite a few of them the talking is probably as important as the needles. They are the kind of people who wouldn't want to go to a psychotherapist or a counsellor, but they use their time with you to talk about things that they can't mention to anyone else. What is more, as you listen to them you start to see some of the patterns in their lives, some of the old behaviours which typically diminish or undermine them, and you start to think of points that might help to loosen the stranglehold of the past. You might even think of building up some countervailing energy. If you are treating someone who complains of painful muscular tension in his neck, for example, because he works very long hours at a desk, but whose life lacks warmth and affection, you might consider using pericardium and heart points even though they have no direct connection to his muscular pain.

And finally, you need a long time for your treatment because you will be designing it as you go. That is, you will check the pulses after each point or set of points in order to see how the energy body has responded to that intervention before you carry on and choose another point. So you have to leave a full hour for each treatment even if you don't always use it, because you have no idea how many points you will need to do until you get a pulse change which you decide is good enough. In fact, that's how you know when to stop. So taking the pulses will be the last thing you do in any treatment.

Now this way of working would be anathema to some acupuncturists I know and respect. It's not only that they wouldn't enjoy doing all that talking nor spending all that time with one patient, they don't really believe in it. For them, the job is to find a well-known and clearly understood diagnosis from among those set out in practically any textbook, to get the needles in quickly and leave them to do their work. These practitioners will take the patient's pulses as part of the initial diagnosis, but may well not do so at the start of subsequent treatments, and certainly won't do so at the end of treatment. What would be the point? They've already done what theory says should be done, so there is actually nothing to learn from any pulse change. And anyway, they get into a kind of rhythm, enjoying the speed and dynamism of constantly moving on to a new patient. One of them once told me that it was like riding a wave, and he hated taking a break because that made him fall off the wave and he sometimes found it hard to get back on again afterwards.

In between these extremes are a number of practitioners who have 20-minute appointments. That works well for those who tend to leave the needles in for about that length of time. They needle patient number one and off they go to another room and take out a set which have been in patient number two for 20 minutes or so. Then they start the third patient and by the time they've got the needles in to that one they're back with the first patient whose needles need to come out – and so on.

There are many options; the point is to find out how you want to work. I've focused on the length of time of your appointments, but I could equally well have looked at the issue of how much you charge for a treatment, the number of rooms you have available, and so on, because they all fit together. If you see one person an hour you'll probably need to charge more than someone who treats three, and that will have an effect on the kind of patients who come to you and the kind of expectations they will have of treatment. In that case, you may well find yourself moving in the direction of the kind of acupuncture which is directed to maintaining health and amplifying potential rather than dealing with physical pain or short-term dysfunction.

Here, to make the point precisely, is a quotation with which some practitioners will agree wholeheartedly and others will find absurd: 'It is not acceptable in Chinese Medicine for pain to be erased while the patient's emotional state declines, for the mobility of the knee to improve while the digestion and circulation deteriorate' (Beinfield and Korngold 1991, p.242).

What do you think? If you have a patient who comes to you complaining of pain and lack of mobility in her knee, would you treat that knee without enquiring about the state of her digestion? And if the knee improves significantly with acupuncture, would you be happy with that even if she is still having digestive problems? Do you think, in fact, that a knee is just a knee – at least sometimes? In other words, that a patient can have a knee problem which has no implications or ramifications for the rest of his mind or body, which is not a sign of some other, more deep seated malaise, but is simply a knee?

This is a complex question and it is not necessarily one to which you want to give a simple answer. But it is worth pondering, especially in the first few years after qualification, because the way you answer it will profoundly influence how you want to work and hence the nature of your practice.

To take one aspect of this, if you see your patient's knee problem as symptomatic of something bigger, then the patient will probably not stop treatment as his knee improves but will tend to keep coming regularly. That's because, through your influence, he will see his treatment as part of a necessary routine which keeps him healthy, like going to the gym or doing yoga. His knee is what brought him into your clinic, but it is not what keeps him there. Now, if you like the prospect of seeing your patients for many years, of doing treatments which are essentially preventive because there is nothing particularly wrong with them at the times they have booked, well and good. But some practitioners would hate it. They much prefer the intensity, I might almost say the drama, of patients who have extreme and urgent conditions and with whom they work in a concentrated way until they are better, and then never see again.

Again, I am not suggesting that one is better than the other in any way; I am simply asking you to consider which of these is the more appealing to you.

It may sound as if this is a bit theoretical. You work the way you do because it is what's possible; the clinic is the only one which had room for you; or you work from home because you don't have enough patients to justify paying rent somewhere else; what you charge is set by what others charge locally; you don't have the time or energy to go back to college, and so on. All perfectly good reasons for doing what you do, but underneath them, like a shark just below the surface, lurks real danger.

Whatever style of acupuncture you use, even if it is at the medical end of the spectrum where a knee is always and only a knee, you cannot escape the fact that a treatment is an interaction between the patient's energy and your own. The two of you are in a room together, your bodies come into contact, and at some level the patient is open to change. Of course we've all seen a few patients who come in order to prove that they've tried everything and nothing works, but the overwhelming majority really want to get better. It isn't the same as a treatment which, after a brief face-to-face diagnosis, consists of taking prescribed drugs every day for a week or a month or a year. Nor is it the same as an operation where, although the patient is in the same room as the surgeon and there is the physical contact, he or she is under anaesthetic. It is this play of and between the two energy bodies which makes an acupuncture treatment qualitatively different from conventional Western medicine and which therefore makes it hard to research using Western medical methodologies; and, which, crucially for you, means that you have to be comfortable with what you are doing in the treatment room.

A tiny example. When I was a student, working under strict supervision, I was treating a woman who liked me but did not much care for my clinical supervisor. One day I marked LI 11 and he came in to check it. He pointed out that my location was wrong, and marked where the point was. I needled it – nothing. I tried again, this time with a different angle – nothing. As you can imagine, I felt such a fool. I couldn't find the point in the first place and then I couldn't even hit it when I'd been told where it was! And how many times could I go on stabbing my poor patient for nothing?

Just then, the supervisor was called out of the room. My patient lifted her head off the couch and said, 'Why don't you needle it where you think it is?' My mouth dropped open. For one thing, it was totally against the rules, and she knew it; and for another, she was effectively saying she trusted me more than him. She saw the doubt on my face, 'Go on,' she said. 'I won't tell.' So I did it, and do you know what? I hit the point. We both knew it.

My supervisor came back into the room and took the patient's pulses. 'Good,' he said. 'That's the change we wanted. You see, LI 11 is much more lateral than you marked it.' The patient and I grinned at each other.

A nice moment, but one to reflect on. What was going on? My supervisor was a very experienced and well-respected practitioner, no question. Did he not know the location of LI 11? Of course he did. In that case, how come I missed it at the correct location and hit it at the incorrect one? The answer to that question lies in the fact that points are not quite what you think they are, at least when you're a beginner, and that hitting them isn't quite what you think it is either. To explain this needs a bit of a digression, but I will come back to the main idea.

You've been taught the correct anatomical location of acupuncture points and indeed it is essential to know them. But they can be misleading. Because the word 'point' means a specific, and usually very tightly defined place, and, because the anatomical locations appear to be very precise, I think it is easy to get the impression that acupuncture points are fixed entities in the body, rather like the place where a tendon attaches to the bone, or an artery runs close to the surface or a nerve exits from the sacrum. But they aren't. They are in, and on, a flow of energy which is in constant movement, and that makes all the difference.

It is quite difficult to really grasp this because, in the West, we see the world as made of things, not processes; objects, not movements. Our language reflects this perception. For example, we have to say 'it' is raining, when there is nothing which could possibly be the 'it'. Strange. We can't say rain is raining, or raining is happening, which would be much nearer what it's really like, because that would be to express the thing as a process. Once you spot this bias in our perceptions and our language, you find it everywhere. So, to ask an impossible question, where does your fist go when you open your hand? There's no answer because 'fist', which seems to be a thing, and therefore can't just disappear, isn't really a thing at all – it's a movement. So, of course, once you've made a new and different movement the old one has happened, and is over.

The reason I've gone into all this is that our language misleads us into thinking that acupuncture points are things. But they aren't. You can't find them by dissection. So what are they? We don't really know, and when we don't know what something is we use analogies to try to understand them.

The best analogy is that points are like eddies or vortices in a river. If you follow the small intestine meridian along from the first point you can see how it works. As the flow of energy hits, and then rolls over the bumps in the bone, an eddy is created; it's just the same in a river. This explains the locations of SI 1 then 2 then 3 then 4 then 5 then 6 (but not 7 – I'll come to that in a moment). Feel it under your finger as you trace the path of the meridian. And, if you think about it, this explains a whole host of points – Liv 3, LI 4, Sp 9, St 36, for example. And, though less obviously, it explains the location of all the upper chest points on the front and back of the body; think of the ribs as a sequence of rock strata, and energy as a river flowing over them (I saw exactly this quite recently on the river Swale at Richmond in Yorkshire). And the same image works for points like Sp 6, where the eddy is created by the junction of different meridians, just as an enormous eddy is created where two or more rivers meet.

But this analogy doesn't work for abdomen point like St 25, or limb points like SI 7 or Pc 6 or Liv 5. What can explain their locations? One answer is to imagine that the meridians are like electric cables and that the points are places where there are switches. The cable runs all round the room and through the walls but, only if you can find the switch and touch it in the right way do you get the light to come on. Quite neat. Another possibility is suggested by the 'glug glug' sound you get when liquid is poured through a narrow funnel. The noise comes from a kind of oscillation. One moment the flow is full, the next it is restricted. Perhaps the same sort of oscillation happens as energy flows along the meridians, and what we call points are simply the places where the flow is strong – so an intervention there has more effect.

Having said this, I must point out that it is all speculation – and it's not even the most puzzling thing about points. What is really mysterious is how a particular point has a very specific effect; how, for example, moxa on Bl 67, but not anywhere else, turns a foetus; or how St 38 eases a stiff and restricted shoulder. All we can say at the moment, maybe all we'll ever be able to say, is 'it just does'.

Now, to get back to the story of needling LI 11 on my patient, my belief is that if my supervisor had needled the point where he marked it he would indeed have hit it. In other words, the point is in different places for different practitioners. Not hugely different, of course, but there is usually quite a bit of leeway within the parameters set down by the anatomical description; enough leeway, at any rate, to make it easy to miss them.

This seems a weird idea. On the famous bronze man, and in countless texts written over many centuries, the point locations are given as absolute, without any doubt or qualification. But if you see these locations as our attempts to express something which is inherently fluid, using a physical model, which isn't a very good representation because it is static, or a language which doesn't give a very accurate description because it is biased towards things, then the idea doesn't seem so strange.

And a crucial aspect of this is whether or not we make our energy available to another person. I'm sure you know what I mean. I'm sure you have felt, in normal daily life, how without moving a muscle you can withdraw yourself from someone who has made a comment which you find hurtful or offensive. And I'm equally sure you know the feeling of opening and extending yourself towards someone who is warm, affectionate and who seems to think you are wonderful. And just as it happens all the time in normal life it happens all the time in the treatment room. And I suspect it happens more, and more powerfully too, because we work in such an intimate way with our patients and their energy bodies.

If my supervisor had needled where he marked the point I suspect he would have got some change, but maybe not a lot. Perhaps the kind of change you get when you push a toboggan whose runners are rusty and pitted; or when you wash up in cool rather than hot water; or when you hoover with worn brushes and a full bag; a kind of slow, inadequate and rather grudging kind of change. By contrast, I think that because my patient and I got on so well her energy was readily available to me and it was willing to come and find my needle, so to speak (as long as

I was near enough to be within reach), and it was happy to respond to what I was asking it to do. It's not so different from dancing. With one person, you keep missing – you head off in different directions, you tread on each other's toes, you have to keep apologising. With another you just seem to flow; each of you somehow knows what the other is up to and finds it just right.

The lesson from all this is not that you have to be friends with all your patients. Inevitably there will be some you feel closer to than others. It is that you need to feel comfortable with the way you practise. This applies to the smallest things as well as the largest. To continue for a moment with the example of point location, if you mark a point where it ought to be and where your rational mind tells you it is, but as you bend down to insert the needle you have a feeling it isn't really there, then do you go ahead and needle? I've done that countless times; quashed the little voice inside me which whispered, 'Er, I'm not so sure about this.' But I don't do it any more. Even if I did hit something which might have been the point, I never got a good pulse change, never saw the patient's face look softer and warmer, never felt that ease spread through the room. Technically it might have been faultless, but actually nothing happened.

I think the same is true with diagnosis. I treated a patient for a few years largely on the basis of a five element diagnosis. She did well with it. Then I took a year off and she went to another practitioner who reached a completely different five element diagnosis and treated her on that basis, also successfully. When I started work again, and the patient came back to me for treatment (for which I was deeply grateful, of course) I was told of the new diagnosis. I could absolutely understand it, it made perfect sense; and I thought to myself, 'Well, I've never been any good at five element acupuncture, so I'll use my colleague's diagnosis, and glad of it.' I started doing points which followed from that diagnosis, points I'd never used on her before, and the results were awful. She came out in a rash, she had headaches she'd never had before, and so on. I was upset and baffled. Surely, surely, now I was using the correct diagnosis she ought to be doing better than when I treated her before, not worse?

It took me ages to understand that a diagnosis isn't an objective truth but a guide. It directs you towards some points and away from others. It implies how many to use and in what order. That's all. And like any guide, like any direction, it will feel right and comfortable and reassuring for some people, and awkward and clumsy and oddly irrelevant to others. What works is what you see in your patient, how you experience his or her energy body and what you believe in. And it's not just that you work better when you're feeling that what you're doing makes sense, it has a profound effect on your own energy body, making it clearer, more coherent and more stable. And your patient will pick up on that. When you're working well and confidently you can feel your patient leaning in towards you, trusting your work and hence making his or her energy body available for change.

I think this principle applies right the way through, from the style of acupuncture you practise, to the place you work, to the amount you charge; everything. If you want to make a success of being an acupuncturist, and to enjoy the work too, you need to be yourself, and you need to trust that that very self, and no other, is what will work best.

CHAPTER 3

KEEPING IT SIMPLE

There is an old saying, 'the best is the enemy of the good', which points to a problem people face in the early years of practice. The saying has multiple meanings. You can take it as meaning, for example, that the benefits of a good treatment are undervalued because they don't look all that great in comparison with the best ones. And the comparison is acute in the early days of practice because you'll have just seen your teachers making remarkable diagnoses, doing wonderful treatments and getting fantastic pulse changes – which doesn't seem to happen in your own treatment room. That can lead you to lose confidence, to think that it's all too difficult, and to believe that you're missing what your patients really need. It's a trap, and one that is all too easy to fall into. For although you may be able to acknowledge that it is simply ridiculous to compare yourself to an expert with years of experience, it's not so easy to stop yourself judging your work against the standards they set, and deciding you've failed. And the truth is that you can help your patients a great deal by doing what you can do at your stage of expertise.

There's another aspect to this as well, and that is the way it influences what you attempt. For all that your teachers have shown you how it can be difficult to reach a diagnosis, and have discussed a range of plausible possibilities before coming to a conclusion, the fact is that when they reach a decision it appears both clear and convincing. Naturally, you think that this is what you must do too. Even if you have to go through a certain amount of agonising and uncertainty, still, when it is time to needle you believe you need to have the sort of clarity they possess. So you believe it is essential to have a coherent diagnosis which will yield treatment principles, and they will have to be prioritised so you can attend to what needs to be done in the right order. Of course, that is a good way to proceed, but it is also another trap. The danger is that in attempting to mimic what skilled practitioners do after many years of experience you make far more mistakes than if you tried to do what is genuinely and realistically within your capabilities, which is another example of the best being the enemy of the good.

Here's an example from my own practice. My patient is a woman in her mid fifties, a warm, smiling, jolly presence whose main complaint is her weight. About five foot four inches high she weighs 17 stone. She's at the point where she's in a vicious circle. She feels bad about her weight so she eats to comfort herself. Exercise is really exhausting so she doesn't do any. As a result, she puts on more weight and feels worse about herself. In general terms it's a pretty familiar pattern. I started out by making a full diagnosis.

I drew up a complicated diagram showing Spleen Qi and Spleen Yang deficiency and their relationship to Kidney Yang deficiency with water overflowing (the oedema of her legs and ankles was especially pronounced). Then I related all these to her other symptoms, such as chronic constipation and occasional migraines, adding in Liver Qi stagnation and possibly Liver Blood deficiency as well. In five element terms I thought her primary imbalance was Earth. So my treatment principles were to clear Damp, support the kidneys, dispel the Liver Qi stagnation, and support the constitutional factor. It looked good. Unfortunately it didn't work.

Just before I go on to explain why, it is worth pausing on the deceptively simple phrase 'didn't work'. You might think the criterion of success in this case is very straightforward: it must be that she starts to lose weight. But what's the timescale? Clearly, it is unlikely that change will happen fast, so how long can you go on before you admit that the treatment doesn't seem to be working? Six sessions, twelve? And how much weight counts as enough to decide the treatment is working: half a stone, a stone, whatever the patient is happy with?

There's no easy answer to these questions and it's an issue with almost every patient, whether you've been in practice for ten weeks or ten years. The reason I raise it here is that I think that the longer you have been in practice the more you are willing to give treatment time to work. There are two parts to this, I think. One is that, after some years and with some successes under your belt, you are not so desperate for quick results. Nor are you so nervous at the thought of being paid by patients who, apparently, have nothing to show for their money.

I well remember one of my teachers saying of a patient, who had been coming regularly for over a year, that there was no sign of any change. 'Why isn't it working?' I asked. 'And how can you keep going?' She smiled and replied that he had an old and deep-seated condition, that she didn't know when it would start to shift, but that when it did she would be there to help. That seems to me to be wise. It speaks of an understanding of how healing can happen, of an inner confidence that the work is good even if there is no immediate evidence of its effects, and of a willingness to trust that the patient who keeps on returning knows that he or she is being helped.

The other point is more familiar to psychotherapists than to acupuncturists. It is that quite often what really needs to change, what is stopping the patient's healing, is not known to him or her. So, of course, it doesn't figure as a complaint, nor as a criterion of how well treatment is working. Here is a good example.

In the first months of my practice a patient came to the clinic, grey and bent and with the pain of a terrible backache. He was a priest... Being in those days eager to 'make people well'...I can tell you that had I known how to treat his back symptomatically I would have done so.

One day I entered the treatment room and saw him sitting fully dressed in the corner. My heart sank; 'He's come to tell me he's stopping treatment,'

I thought, and yet, with curiosity, I noticed he was looking wonderful, radiant even. Sure enough, he said 'Meriel, I have come to tell you I am stopping treatment but I want you to know that acupuncture has cured me. I didn't tell you when I came for treatment of my greatest grief... I didn't tell you that in recent years I had lost the ability to pray, and have lived in such pain... Last night I dreamed that God was speaking to me. He said, 'Don't be concerned about your back, I am with you.' My back feels fine today. (Darby 2003, p.34)

It's moving, isn't it, to hear about that level of healing?

Which brings me back to my overweight patient. I knew treatment wasn't working not simply because she didn't lose any weight, but because I sensed no response from her energy body. Her pulses responded a bit to the needles but by the following treatment had dropped back to where they had been before. More significantly, there was no real change in her. She still presented a cheery face to the world, still walked with the same waddle, still had an unexpected look in her eyes, one which was quite fierce and sharp. And there was more to it than that. I felt that I hadn't seen her, not really, and that until I did her energy body would remain inaccessible, untouched. So I decided that for the next few treatments I would drop my complicated diagnosis, spend a bit more time talking to her, not so much for the content of the conversation but more to try and tune in to her energy body and what it really needed, and then do whatever felt appropriate in the moment.

I am still astonished, although I have seen it many times now, how if you unlock one thing you unlock everything. I did a very simple treatment, one I'm not sure I could have arrived at through any of the systems of diagnosis I know. I'm not even sure I could explain how I arrived at it. Anyway, I needled Ren 4, then Ht 7.

The next week, something had shifted. She looked different, and she told me that she had noticed a change in her ankles. At work, she always took her shoes off whenever she could because they cut into her flesh where it overflowed the tops of her shoes. But one day she'd been at her desk for a whole morning and had forgotten to take them off because they weren't hurting. And indeed, her legs did look a bit less distended and they were a better colour too. Then, as we talked, a whole story came out about what had happened to her when she was a teenager and a young adult, a story she'd never told properly before because she hadn't realised its significance in her life. It seemed that the two things, starting to come back to her right shape and weight and telling the story of a very difficult time in her life, were both part of the same process of releasing something that had been pent up and contained within her, and which had distorted her physically and emotionally. At the time of writing the process continues. She has lost only a little weight, but it seems to be better distributed in her body. Her other symptoms have cleared up too and she feels much better in herself.

The point of this example is that I failed with the kind of comprehensive diagnosis I was taught to do, but succeeded with something much simpler, much more provisional and considerably less dogmatic.

It isn't hard to see how this works. It's partly that once I'd let go of all that stuff about organs and pathogens I was able to see her energy body more clearly; an instance of seeing the wood for the trees. It's also that the complexity of my initial diagnosis provided me with so many ways to go wrong. If treatment wasn't working was it because I should have tonified Kidney first rather than cleared Damp? And if I was right to try and clear Damp first did I go wrong by dispersing Sp 6 and 9 when it would have been better to tonify Sp 3 and St 36 – and so on and so on. The possibilities of error are practically endless.

The sheer rationality of a clear diagnosis can mislead in other ways too. If, as it suggests so powerfully, you know exactly what you are doing then you might as well get on with it. Your diagnosis tells you, for example, to nourish Heart and Kidney Yin, clear Empty Heat and nourish Blood, but it doesn't tell you how long to take over it. The temptation, especially in the early years of practice when you are so keen that your patients show quick signs of improvement, is to try to do all, or most of it, at once. That cuts out the possibility of accurate feedback. If you've done two or three things in one treatment, and it hasn't worked, then you have no idea what to change next time.

Actually, the problem is just as acute, though it doesn't seem so at first, if the treatment was a success; for then, because you can't go on doing exactly the same treatment for ever, you won't know how to maintain the success. I know a very experienced practitioner who is so certain that his initial diagnosis won't be good enough, and that he will need plenty of feedback before he is confident of being able to help, that he won't agree to take on a new patient unless he or she commits to six treatments. An extreme position perhaps, but one that gives full weight to the need for flexibility, for taking time to learn, and for designing early treatments which can provide unambiguous guidance for the future. In order to achieve these aims you don't have to go as far as he does, or as I went with my overweight patient when I abandoned the whole of my initial diagnosis, but you do have to be a bit careful and even a bit ruthless with yourself. And when you are recently qualified that almost always means doing less than you really want to do and making the treatment simpler than the one you first thought of. And it also means refusing to listen to that little voice that may whisper in your ear the terrible temptation, 'The patient won't think it's worth coming unless I do some more points.'

So far I've talked about keeping it simple from the point of view of the practitioner, as a way of making sure you don't overreach yourself. But it is also important to think about it from the point of view of the patient and of his or her energy body. You are trying to facilitate change, to steer the body, so to speak, away from the well-trodden path which has led it into its current predicament and onto a new and unfamiliar route to health.

You will be dealing both with an opponent and an ally. Part of your patient, unconsciously of course, will resent the effort needed and will be attached to the benefits of his or her current state, however disabling. On the other hand, as countless tales of recovery from apparently incurable conditions testify, there is a reserve of strength even in those with very severe illness, and there is in all of us a deep impulse to heal.

Both the opponent and the ally need to be respected. The opponent can be mollified, basically, by not asking it to do too much at once. To some extent that's because its cooperation is usually somewhat grudging, but more because change genuinely takes energy and effort. Don't forget that your treatment will make demands on a system which is probably already struggling to manage normal life. It also helps if you can also appeal to what it likes best. Does it lean towards Yin or Yang? Would it prefer, therefore, the bracing quality of Du points or the comfort of Ren ones? Another possibility is to stick with the basic command points until you feel that the patient's system is able to respond readily to the needles.

As for the ally, the best approach is to play to its strengths. It is so easy when hearing a tale of ill health or dysfunction, when taking pulses which are alarmingly low or when looking at a tongue which speaks of multiple disorders, to focus on pathology and to think all the time about how to tackle what is wrong. In that case you can lose sight of the option of amplifying the patient's strengths. In Western medical terms, it is building up the immune system rather then eliminating pathogens.

In my early days of training I was instructed to see my patient as he or she could be, should be, in full and abundant health. It wasn't altogether easy and anyway it seemed a bit of a luxury when I was cudgelling my brains to come up with a plausible diagnosis, so I soon forgot about it. Until, that is, I'd been in practice for many years and realised that it was exactly what I was doing after all. It's not hard, and it does give you some options you wouldn't have thought of otherwise. My guess is that this is exactly what happened to the priest with a bad back. I think that his practitioner, perhaps without quite realising it (she wrote, 'had I known how to treat his back symptomatically I would have done so'), treated what we call his soul or his spirit, that part of him which had taken him into the priesthood in the first place, and by strengthening it had brought about the change. Maybe the same is true of my overweight patient too. Certainly, it became clear to me that her strength was a Yin kind of strength and that she had, as we say, a big heart; which does suggest Ren points and Ht 7.

Whether you choose to pacify the opponent or support the ally, your treatment needs to convey an unambiguous message; otherwise the ally will try to do everything, and fail, and the opponent will be able to avoid doing anything at all. Keeping it simple doesn't just mean using fewer points than you might be tempted to do but using combinations of points which convey a clear, simple idea to the energy body. I'll illustrate this with a couple of recent examples where students have done treatments which seemed to me to be muddled, and hence ineffective.

One patient was being treated, long term, for the effects of Hepatitis B; short term he was suffering from insomnia and palpitations. The student tonified Liv 1 and 3 and then

Ht 9. You can see what she had in mind. Liv 1, although normally used for disorders of the lower jiao, is also the Wood point of the Liver so it will have delivered a boost to its energy. The source point would have done the same. Then Ht 9, as the Jing Well point is often used to clear Heat, but it is also the tonification point for the heart, so it would have provided a stimulus to the energy of the heart. The practitioner probably hoped that this would help it to recover its normal rhythm, thereby stopping the palpitations and perhaps relieving the insomnia too. However, putting these points together conveys a very mixed message; Liv 1 and 3 suggest that the energy of the liver is weak and has to be strengthened, but then, immediately, its energy is taken away to support the heart. That is likely to leave the patient's energy body confused, unclear how to respond. 'I can't do both,' you can imagine it saying, 'so which do you want me to do?' And of course the treatment gives no answer to that perfectly reasonable question.

Another example comes from treating a channel problem, specifically numbness in the patient's legs. The student's diagnosis was Damp, with an underlying Qi deficiency. So he needled Sp 6, and 9, then added Ki 7, all with even technique, and then tonified Liv 3. Individually all these points might help; the first three all clear Damp and the last one will have a powerful effect in clearing the channel. But the combination is messy. If the top priority is to clear Damp, then it would have been better to have used the Spleen points and added St 36 and left it at that. Or, if it is more important to clear the channels, then it would be better to take the energy down the leg with points on Yang meridians and back up again with points on Yin ones; and it is surely easier to envisage energy flowing more freely if the points are on paired channels, Bladder and Kidney or Gallbladder and Liver, but not a mixture of the two.

One way of arriving at simple treatments, especially when you feel a little uncertain, is to remind yourself that what you are doing when you use needles and moxa is moving energy (and, with moxa, amplifying it to some extent). You might be torn between smoothing Liver Qi stagnation and nourishing Liver Blood – quite a common dilemma. Or, if you practise five element acupuncture, you might find you can't make up your mind whether the patient is Fire or Earth. What to do? 'Both,' might seem to be the answer that covers the bases, but it'll probably lead you into doing a complicated and confusing treatment. There is a well-known saying in chess, 'In the beginner's mind there are many possibilities; in the expert's, very few.' That's it, exactly. You need to cut away the reams of possibilities so you are left with very few, and a good way of doing that is to go back to the basic issue of moving energy. Listening to your patient, looking at him or her, taking the pulses, looking at the tongue, simply ask yourself, 'What energy needs moving?' and then, 'Where does it need to move to?' You'll be amazed at the clarity of the answers that occur to you.

After all, we normally classify Qi in a limited number of ways; either by its organ, by its location, or its quality. And there are a limited number of directions it can move in. It can be encouraged to flow from inside to outside, as when clearing Wind Cold or Damp Heat in the lungs.

It can be stimulated to flow from top to bottom, or vice versa, as when we treat Liver Yang rising or Spleen Qi sinking. Finally, deficiency can be strengthened by moving Qi from where there is enough, as when we use tonification points, and excess can be dispersed. It's a bit shocking to think that it can all be summed up so brutally briefly, and although there is scope for enormous subtlety within this framework, the bare bones do provide a fair and useful description of what we do.

So what I'm suggesting is that if you're getting over-complicated, or over-worried in your diagnoses, then it may well be that you are finding it difficult to go from the patient's signs and symptoms straight to decisions expressed in the technical language of syndromes, or whatever other diagnostic categories you use. For some of you, it will be because those categories seem a little artificial, theoretical. For others, it may be leading you into trying to puzzle out the answer as if the patient were a sudoku with one correct answer. Then again, it may just be that you are on a bad run, as they say of sportsmen, and your confidence is low. Whatever the source of the difficulty, it really helps to go back to the very basics.

Using those basics will lend a particular quality to your diagnoses and treatments, one which I know I appreciate as a patient, and that is the quality of an invitation. If the practitioner is simply trying to move one type of energy, then it feels like an offer, a suggestion. 'How about this?' you can imagine the treatment as asking, then adding, 'I think you might be more comfortable over there.' And if that's right, or at least right enough, the body can pick it up and respond; and if it isn't, then it can simply be ignored. By contrast, complicated treatments have an air of authority, an air of demanding compliance – they remind me of my school P.E. teacher – and I don't think I am alone in having an instinctive resistance to that kind of thing.

Many years ago now, when I was in my last six months at college, we had to visit acupuncturists in their clinics and sit in on their treatments. The word got around, of course, as to which ones were the most interesting and which ones were best avoided. I had to do my last day with one of the latter because everyone else was full. And I could see what my colleagues meant. With the odd exception, all the practitioner did with each patient was the two source points on a pair of meridians, LI 4 and Lu 9, for example, or the two tonification points, say, Bl 67 and Ki 7. It took me a while to get beyond being unimpressed. In fact, the atmosphere in the treatment room was delightful; in fact, the pulse changes he got were excellent; in fact, his patients all reported that they were doing well; in fact, they all looked better after the treatment. It was a huge teaching. He wasn't working in this way because he was incompetent or limited, but because he had found a way to work simply and effectively. Working in that way is not for everyone. But finding your own version of his simplicity is a wonderful route from novice to expert.

CHAPTER 4

PULSES

Just as there are many different styles of acupuncture so there are many different styles of pulse-taking. In fact, the two go together. In Traditional Chinese Medicine (TCM) where the pulses are normally used for diagnosis only, the practitioner will take them at the start of the treatment, but will not normally take them again in the same session. That is because once they have been used to decide what to do, to clear Damp or move Liver Qi stagnation for example, then what else could the practitioner learn from taking them again? By contrast, in some forms of five element acupuncture, the pulses are not used at all for diagnosis, which depends on the patient's colour, odour and so on, but are used to provide feedback. Hence the practitioner will normally check them after each point, or set of points, to find out how the patient has responded.

Then there is another kind of disparity. In TCM, the pulse is said to have a number of qualities like choppy, wiry and slippery, and the practitioner needs to be able to identify them in order to reach a diagnosis. By contrast, practitioners of most other styles of acupuncture do not even attempt to classify the pulses in this way. They look simply for improvement; whatever the pulse was like at the start of a treatment they want it to be better at the end. If asked to describe this 'better' they will say things like, it feels softer (or rounder or stronger) – which implies that originally it was hard (or sharp or weak) – descriptions which they do not use to tell them what to do but simply to provide a baseline against which treatment can be measured.

I can sum up these differences by saying that pulse-taking in TCM does not involve comparison, whereas in most other forms of acupuncture it usually does.

This can be very confusing if you have been taught by people who practise different styles of acupuncture. After all, it is hard enough to learn to take pulses accurately without having to worry about what kind of pulse-taking you should be doing, let alone when you should be doing which. But I think that there is a way of thinking about pulse-taking which can combine the best of both styles and help you to improve both your skills and your treatments.

I'll start by saying something about the advantages of each of them. One of the best things about the comparison style (as I will call it from now on, to distinguish it from the TCM style) is that it is much less demanding. All it requires is that you register what the pulse feels like. It isn't even necessary to put that feeling into words, but if you want to do so then whatever language you choose will do fine – a bit squashy, or flickering, or wobbly, are all perfectly good descriptions, even though they appear in no acupuncture text, because you know what you mean by them and because they give you a clear baseline. So it will be easy to tell if, after treatment, the pulse is less squashy or more regular or solid, and therefore to know if the treatment has had the effect you wanted.

By contrast, for a TCM diagnosis you will need to decide, at least, on the depth, width, strength, rate, rhythm and shape of the pulse (and of individual pulses if they show marked differences from the rest) and that is quite a challenge. Most simply, and probably most crucially, the main benefit of this style is to distinguish between full and empty conditions, because that will tell you whether to tonify or disperse.

This is no trivial matter. I firmly believe that doing one when you should be doing the other is the single biggest error you can make; it is certainly the biggest single error I make.

When I have done a treatment which did not help, or sometimes even aggravated the patient's condition, it is usually because I tonified when I should have dispersed, or vice versa. And, almost another way of saying the same thing, TCM pulse-taking will tell the practitioner when it is necessary to clear pathogens before doing anything else. I hate to think how many times I tonified Spleen or Kidney or even Sanjiao when I should have cleared Damp first.

So much for the main advantages of each style. But, as with any system, it is worth looking not just at how good it is when it is used properly but how good it is when it isn't used very well. Given that none of us is perfect and that we all make mistakes, especially when we are learning, what kind of errors do we fall into with each of these styles of pulse-taking, and how serious are they?

Because the TCM system demands a good deal of discrimination and precision it tends towards one particular, and quite fundamental kind of error. What can happen is that you spend so long crouched over the pulse trying to decide if, for example, it is really thin, or weak, or sinking, or all three, and whether or not the Lung pulse is a little fuller than the rest, that you miss their overall message; in this example, that the patient's energy is depleted. What's more, all this discrimination tends to set your mental process into overdrive as you worry away at whether a pulse is wiry or tight (at the same time as you can't help thinking that you're not entirely sure you remember what the difference between the two of them is supposed to be). And, of course, if you are in your head you can't be in your fingertips at the same time – so while you are busy thinking about the pulse you are missing the information it is offering up to you. I well remember teaching a group of newly qualified practitioners. We all took a patient's pulses which, to me, screamed of excess, probably Blood stagnation, but when I asked the students what they had discovered all but a few of them reported solemnly that Bladder and Kidney were a bit weak. That's not seeing the wood for the trees.

The main danger of the comparison approach is that you get sloppy. There are many ways this can happen. One is that you take a quick first impression, registering one key characteristic, they're all a bit fast, and leave it at that. Then, after a few points, when you check the pulses again and decide that they've slowed down nicely, you're satisfied with the change when actually there was so much more to discover and to do. More dangerous, perhaps, is the trap you fall into when you take pulses which are complicated in some way, with disparities in the strength and shape of individual pulses, and you don't bother to investigate properly, thinking it's good enough to say to yourself something like, they're a bit funny, hmmm, not together somehow. Then, even if you do get a change for the better you don't really know what has changed, and so you can't learn much from the treatment. And, of course, if the points you've chosen don't seem to help, you have no clue as to what to try next.

Having set out the dangers of each approach, it's easy to see how they can be avoided. If you have learned TCM and practise in that way, then you can simply ask yourself, what's the first thing my fingertips pick up from these pulses? What jumps onto them, demanding attention? By the way, rather than just asking, 'What do I notice?', it really is a good idea to specify your fingertips because that helps to keep your attention there; and that, in turn will help you to refine and develop your skills.

For those who use the comparison style it is helpful to be aware of some of the categories of TCM pulse-taking in order to get more than a baseline from your initial reading. It's not that you have to know, let alone recognise, the conventional 28 pulse qualities, but if you have a pulse which comes up to your fingertips clearly and forcefully, what some people call a pulse that's in your face, it really is a great question to ask yourself, is this pulse floating or not? In other words, if you press down on it, does it stay strong, maybe even feel stronger, or does it collapse and sort of disappear? You don't have to have been trained in

TCM for this to be useful information. If it stays strong then you are definitely dealing with excess of some kind; so the test of a good treatment will be that the pulse gets a little deeper and less forceful – 'weaker' isn't quite the right word because it suggests a kind of feebleness – as the excess is dispersed. On the other hand, if the pulse is floating and has no real inner strength, then you do want it to feel stronger after treatment. It may not be as prominent, indeed you hope it won't be, but it will have a kind of resilience and robustness that it lacked before.

I want to turn now to the issue of taking pulses throughout the treatment, or at the end, or both. Whatever style of acupuncture you practise, I cannot see any argument for not taking the pulses at the end of a treatment. You need the feedback; it's how you learn anything. And in the vast majority of cases the pulses give excellent, fast and objective feedback. The pulses are not trying to be nice or good, they don't need you to like them or to understand how hard their life is, they don't have to challenge whatever you say; all ways in which feedback from your patient can be distorted.

Think of pulse changes along a spectrum. At one end is the most wonderful, amazing change you've felt in a very long time; confirmation, surely, that your diagnosis was exactly right and that you can proceed with confidence in future. At the other end of the spectrum the pulses get significantly worse from treatment. That is, whatever quality you noticed as your benchmark, for example that they were tight or too full, has become more noticeable, and there may be an extra dimension of awfulness too. A sure sign that you have not understood at all, and probably that you are doing the exact opposite of what the patient needs.

Most of our treatments lie between these two extremes, and here we learn even more. Imagine you are a TCM practitioner and that in last week's treatment you cleared Wind Heat in a patient. The pulses slowed and felt softer and fuller. Good. And the patient comes back this week and reports that he has felt much better, and hasn't been so aware of the hot head of which he had complained, though it hasn't completely gone away. Very good. You decide to do the same treatment again. This time there is no real change from the pulses. That is absolutely invaluable information. Now you know that you have dealt with the Wind Heat, and you also know that there is something else going on as well which you need to diagnose in order to make further progress.

And apart from all these sensible arguments, there is a kind of arrogance about not taking the pulses at the end of a treatment. It seems to say that you know you have done a good job, every time, so there's no need to check. No one is that good.

The same basic argument applies to taking the pulses during a treatment too (though I feel a good deal less strongly about this). To take a simple example, many traditions consider 20 minutes as a kind of standard length of time for needles to be left in, and practitioners in these traditions organise their work around it. Of course, there is nothing wrong with that, but I can't help thinking that it misses two obvious opportunities to improve what they do.

One is that the needles may have done their work in much less than the 20 minutes. Some say that it doesn't matter if the needles stay in after they have done their work, because then they aren't doing anything at all. That isn't my experience. Generalising, if the needles are left in after the patient's energy has changed, I find that their effect seems to get steadily diluted. It is as if the energy body gets the message that the change it has managed just isn't enough, that more is required, and so it tries to carry on doing it. But as it attempts to squeeze more change out of a tiring system it begins to deplete that system, and that can leave the patient so drained that all the gains of the initial work are lost, and the good undone. It's a bit like asking someone to run five miles, which they manage fine, but at the end of the race telling them they have to run it again.

If you check the pulses regularly they will tell you when to take the needles out, because while they are still working the pulses will continue to improve. Then there will be a period where there is no change, and that's the time to take them out.

Another reason for taking the pulses during a treatment is that you want to know if that treatment is working. If it isn't, then you can take the needles out, think again, and try something different. I remember doing a treatment during my last weeks as a student when I did a couple of points and the pulses got worse. I turned to my teacher and asked him what to do. He replied, memorably, if hot doesn't work, try cold. In other words, at least you know what doesn't work, so try the opposite. I did, and everything improved. Even now, I can I remember the relief of turning round what had promised to be a rotten treatment. And the lesson I took away from it is that I didn't actually know whether a particular point, or set of points was going to work in the way I intended, so I'd better check. Twenty years later, I still do.

Whenever you choose to take the pulses, and however many times you take them during a treatment you want to gather as much information from them as you can, and there is one way of doing this which, in my opinion, is supreme. That is to take a moment to predict how they will change after you've needled. Like most of us, I have a natural bias towards believing that my ideas are good ones, and this can lead me to accept a pulse change as an improvement when it really is nothing of the sort. The kind of things I say to myself are, well…it's a bit better, or, I'd like a little more but I think that's probably enough. But if I make myself predict what pulse change I am expecting before I needle, that is a foolproof way of making sure I don't cheat. If I don't get the change I predicted it means I haven't done what I planned, that I haven't understood something, and that I need to think again. Crucial information.

Predicting a change is also a great way of combining the best of both styles of pulse-taking. Having to say in what way the pulses will change certainly makes sure you have a benchmark, and it tends to make it a tighter one too. It also forces you to be specific about your diagnosis. Even at the simplest level, this is invaluable. Think, for example, of the predictions you'll make on the basis of your chosen needle technique. Over-simplifying a bit, if you choose to disperse, you expect the pulses to calm, soften, drop in strength and volume. What if they don't? Maybe what you took as fullness is really just a front and actually the patient is weak. Similarly, if you tonify, you expect the pulses to lift, to become stronger and fuller; what if they get stronger but also thinner? In either case, the disparity between what you predicted and what you got will push you to reconsider your initial diagnosis.

To take a more subtle example, I worked recently with a student who diagnosed Blood deficiency in his patient and chose to needle St 36, Liv 8 and Ht 7. Perfectly plausible. I asked him how he expected the pulses to change. I hope they'll all get fuller and stronger, he replied. Again, it made sense. But if, instead, he'd chosen to needle St 36 and Sp 6 with a prediction that all the pulses would become fuller and stronger, not simply those of Stomach and Spleen, he'd have learned a lot more. If that was indeed what he got, then he'd know that Spleen Blood deficiency was probably the most important weakness. If he didn't get that change then he could try Liv 8 and Bl 18 to see if it was really an underlying Liver Blood deficiency, or perhaps Ht 7 and Pc 6 for Heart Blood deficiency. The point is that getting into the habit of predicting a pulse change will lead you to devise treatments that give you more and better feedback, and that in turn will make your treatments more accurate and more powerful.

There are two more aspects of pulse-taking which usually go unnoticed when you are a student but which you have time to explore when you are no longer so anxiously learning the basics. The first is touch. There is so much information communicated through touch. You will, whether you know it or not, be sending powerful and complex messages to your patients simply by the way you touch them; and their reaction to that touch will send clear messages back to you. And don't forget that touch on a pulse can carry an extra charge when, as is often the case, it is the first time that you and your patient are literally in touch with each other.

Many practitioners pick up the patient's hand in order to take the pulse. It's a kind of a handshake, and we all know how much information that conveys. A loose and floppy handshake can speak of a person who lacks the confidence to bring their presence to your attention. And that isn't quite the same as the floppy handshake of someone who makes no effort to meet you properly, who is indifferent to your presence. At the other extreme there are those whose handshake is too firm, even a little bullying, as if insisting on a kind of dominance or superiority.

So, what message do you think you are communicating by the way you pick up your patient's hand to take the pulses? Is it, I am sympathetic and caring? or, I am busy and efficient? or, I am just doing this in a strictly neutral, professional way? If you haven't thought about it before, it is worth mulling it over and even asking a few people if it is indeed what they feel from your touch, because the chances are that you do it so unconsciously and so automatically that it might not be quite as you think. And once you know, you can change it if you want, as I have done. My touch used to be cloying, lingering, a bit rich and thick, too pressingly caring and smothering for many people's taste. So I learned to make it crisper, cleaner and clearer.

This raises another aspect of the issue, which is that not all patients will like the same kind of touch. Do you pick up the hand differently with different people? Most practitioners don't, mainly because it has never occurred to them to do so. But if we want our patients to be at ease in our presence, and to be open to what acupuncture can provide, it makes sense to touch each one of them in a way that he or she finds comfortable; certainly if a patient shrinks from our touch and closes down against us then that will drastically reduce the potential of the treatment. It's not difficult to adjust your touch. It is one of those things that you don't do only because you don't realise it can be done.

Nor is it just a matter of making your patient feel comfortable. I think it is part of any thorough diagnosis. That is, you are trying to understand how your patient's energy works, the ways in which it typically struggles, and the kind of circumstances which make it easier or harder for it to cope. Knowing how a person likes to be touched tells you a great deal about the overall state of his or her energy. Those with Liver Qi stagnation, for example, will not normally care for a soft and slow touch; they are too impatient for that. On the other hand, those whose Spleen Qi is weak will usually like it because it will speak of the kind of support which is hard for them to provide for themselves.

Some practitioners don't pick up the hand when taking pulses. What I've said above still applies, though it is more subtle. There is a world of difference between the way different practitioners palpate the artery; some pause for quite a long time before pressing down with the fingertips, as if waiting for something in order to start (for the patient to get used to the touch? Just out of habit?) while others start quickly: some linger on the pulses while others dart from one to the other, comparing them, and so on. All these convey different messages, and they are all the more potent for being unspoken.

Above and beyond all this, or perhaps I should say at a deeper level, is simply the power of being touched. It's enshrined in our language. To say that we are touched by someone or something is to report on a powerful inner experience, and one which we cherish, even when the events which gave rise to it may have been sad or even tragic. To be touched evokes the best in us; whether it is gratitude for a kindly act, an impulse to help those in need, or a delighted recognition of the power for good which resides in our fellow human beings. If, when you take a patient's pulse, you touch in this sense of the word, then you will have done something to alleviate his or her condition. And for some patients, those who are lonely, isolated, deprived of loving contact, this may be more valuable than anything you can do with your needles. Here is a story, told by a doctor at Yale Medical School, which makes the point perfectly.

Yeshi Dhonden...takes her hand, raising it in both of his own... His eyes are closed as he feels for her pulse. In a moment he has found the spot... All the power of the man seems to have been drawn down into this one purpose... I cannot see their hands joined in a correspondence that is exclusive, intimate, his fingertips receiving the voice of her sick body through the rhythm and throb she offers at her wrist. All at once I am envious – not of him...but of her. I want to be held like that, touched so, received. And I know that I, who have palpated a hundred thousand pulses, have not felt a single one.

At last Yeshi Dhonden...turns to leave... As he nears the door, the woman raises her head and calls out to him in a voice at once urgent and serene. 'Thank you, doctor,' she says, and touches with her other hand the place he had held on her wrist, as though to recapture something that had visited there. (Dass and Gorman 1992, pp.119–120)

If, in your normal daily work, you remember that pulse-taking can have this power, then even if you think you'll never be as good as Yeshi Dhonden, the quality of your own pulse-taking will change dramatically for the better.

CHAPTER 5

MISTAKES

The practice of acupuncture is a life-long journey of exploration and discovery, so you will go on learning more and more about it until the day you decide to stop working. You may learn some new forms of diagnosis and treatment, or some specialisms like treating children; but mostly what you'll learn is what you were taught at college, except that you'll be finding out how to do it more quickly, more accurately, more powerfully and with a wider range of conditions. You already know enough to work well, so what you need to learn next is how to work better. To some extent you can get that from courses and books and from talking to colleagues, but much of your learning will come from making mistakes.

If you are to became a better practitioner it is absolutely essential that you make mistakes. The deep lessons, the ones you never forget, are those where you feel dreadful about something you've done and you know without a shadow of doubt that you will never do it again. In other words, although it doesn't feel like it at the time, mistakes really are helpful because you'll learn far more from them than from any successful treatment.

Before I go on to talk about the kinds of mistakes you will make (because we all do) and the ways in which you can recover from them (because we all need to), I want to explain why it is that you make mistakes. After all, when you stop to think about it, it is a bit strange. For example, not long ago and with a bunch of eager students all around me, I announced I was going to needle Bl 60. I bent over the patient's ankle and did it (rather nicely if I say so myself). I definitely got the point. As I was straightening up in order to explain exactly how to locate Bl 60, one of the students, God bless him, pointed out that I was on the wrong side of the leg and that in fact I had just needled Ki 3. I haven't blushed like that in a long time. And I am certain I won't make that particular mistake again.

There was a particular cause of that mistake at that time on that day, but it is more interesting to look at the three basic reasons why this sort of thing happens. If, the next time you make a mistake, you notice which of these was the cause of your own error, you'll learn a lot about your strengths and weaknesses as a practitioner.

The first is to do with confidence. There is the familiar problem of self-fulfilling prophecies; those who don't think they can find a particular point, or tell if a pulse is choppy, or see colours in a patient's face, will get flustered when they try to do so, and often talk themselves out of what they first noticed (which was probably correct). They start to doubt themselves, to spend their time in the treatment room worrying about their own abilities rather than concentrating on the patient, and they end up feeling hopeless and inadequate. It is no wonder that their treatments tend to be ineffective.

The opposite, that is over-confidence, is even worse. Practitioners who are so sure of their diagnosis that they keep on treating on that basis and ignore evidence to the contrary: the skin rash that doesn't clear up, or even gets worse; the periods that keep on being heavy and painful; the migraines which come as often as they did – these practitioners are positively dangerous. They say things like, well, it's because the patient doesn't come often enough, as if more of what didn't work the first time will do the trick. Or, if the patient's symptoms get worse, they suggest that it's a temporary dip, a necessary stage on the road to recovery. Well, it might be. There is indeed such a thing as a healing crisis, a predictable, highly specific and temporary aggravation of symptoms. It is quite unusual in my experience, though it does happen. In treating chronic asthma, for example, you may well get a brief recurrence of childhood eczema. But unless the practitioner has predicted that kind of occurrence with some accuracy, then you can be pretty sure it isn't a stage of healing but simply the result of poor treatment. Fundamentally, the problem with this kind of over-confidence is that the practitioner doesn't learn, and so never rectifies his or her mistakes or gets better at the work.

The second reason you might make mistakes is that you have some sort of issue with your patient. There is a lot more about this in Chapter 6, but for now I just want to give a couple of examples of how it might apply to you.

Have you ever looked at your appointments for the day, seen that a particular patient is coming, and had a sinking feeling in your stomach? That's it. Or perhaps, at the end of a treatment, you find yourself reluctant to make another appointment for him or her, maybe even suggesting that it would be a good idea to have a few weeks or months without treatment, when you're not completely sure that is in the patient's best interests. That's it too.

And what about the opposite? Do you have any patients for whom you make a special effort – perhaps you wear nicer clothes or you take time to put on make-up or comb your hair? Maybe you give them more time, find yourself being more sympathetic than usual, or catch yourself telling them about yourself and your own life. All danger signs.

If this kind of thing is happening then you won't be able to see that person clearly nor treat with accuracy. You are being attracted to, or repelled by, something that is nothing to do with your patient, nothing to do with who he or she really is. You are simply seeing some aspect of your own nature, an aspect which you don't fully recognise or accept in yourself. It is well understood in the psychoanalytical literature, where it is called projection. The idea is that you project your own unacknowledged qualities onto the patient, much as a film is projected onto a screen. If I am not aware of my own selfishness, for example, then when I get a glimpse of it in someone else I will react strongly to that person, may even hate him for what I can't bear to acknowledge in myself; and that will certainly make it impossible to treat him properly.

The third basic cause of mistakes is having doubts about acupuncture itself. If you're reading this book you will be tremendously enthusiastic about this form of medicine, and will have embraced it with a genuine passion. Almost all of us feel the same way. Acupuncture seems to us to be a source of profound wisdom; a wisdom, what is more, which is generally ignored in Western culture. But later, after qualification, doubts can creep in. It may be because when you're on your own you can't seem to get the results you used to get at the college clinical; it may be because you come across conditions that don't seem to respond to treatment; it may be because (and it has happened to most of us) a patient has had an adverse reaction to one of your treatments and that has shaken you. Perhaps you have had some patients who you thought were doing well but they didn't come back. Or you might be affected by research which seems to have shown that dummy needles (inserted not at acupuncture points) work just as well as real ones. Is the whole thing just placebo, you ask yourself? Am I wasting my time and energy trying to reach an accurate diagnosis, sensing pulse qualities and worrying about which points would be best if it doesn't actually matter where I insert the needles?

If you bring these doubts into the treatment room then you will be undermining your work. Whatever you do, do it fully. If you're not sure about tongue diagnosis, for example, and wonder if it really is accurate, then read books about it, go to a workshop, talk to colleagues and make up your mind. But don't do it half-heartedly and without conviction. If need be, stop doing it for a while and see if you miss it. If you do, then pick it up again; if not, then maybe it's best to give it up. You don't have to do everything and you certainly don't have to be good at everything.

Now for the kinds of mistakes you may make. Here's an example from my own practice. A woman of 32 comes to see me. She is obviously very bright and dynamic, and equally obviously she is currently very depleted. She complains primarily of dizziness (though there is no visual disturbance) and a feeling that her head doesn't belong on her shoulders. She gets dizzy even when she turns over in bed at night; she has fallen a few times, very suddenly, and sometimes has the disturbing sensation of losing control of her body. Her doctor diagnosed labyrinthitis and prescribed antibiotics, which made no difference at all. She has been off work for over two months from a job she loves, and has had to give up driving. She tried working from home but finds that she can't concentrate, and that her memory is poor. Additionally, she has a strong burning sensation before and after, but not during, urination. She has a cheesy white discharge most days, but only manages to move her bowels every third day or so. Her lower abdomen is distinctly cold and she looks pale. Her pulses are weak and thin and her tongue is dark and a bit swollen with a dry whitish coat.

Well it's quite a mish-mash, to me at any rate. There are intimations of Blood Xu or Stagnation, or both, of Wind (but why?) of Damp, of both Heat and Cold. I suspect her constitutional element is Earth, but then when I start to think of syndromes, Kidney and Liver ones spring to mind.

Moxa ought to be helpful to her overall depletion, but would it aggravate the burning urination? Is she so weak that if I try to expel Cold or Damp I might leave her even more enfeebled?

Well, I decided to use mainly Earth points because she was clearly depleted, and because I thought they would help to pull energy down from her head. After a few treatments I added moxa, cautiously at first, but it seemed to suit her – at any rate the burning got no worse. Later I tried tonifying Blood with Bl 17 and 20 but she didn't do so well the following week so I dropped that idea. She got better slowly and after about nine or ten treatments was well enough to drive her car and go back to work. But after a few more treatments, and certainly before she was fully recovered, she stopped coming.

I've thought about her a lot because I felt, and still feel, that I failed her. She had been unwell in all sorts of ways for many years. The dizziness was a kind of final collapse of the system, and I was sure that treatment was an opportunity for her to get over a host of problems and to be better than she had been for years. And I am sure that if my diagnosis had been more accurate she'd have carried on coming. For example, looking back over my notes, I can hardly believe that I never used St 40 to clear Phlegm, and never needled Liv 3 or GB 43 to bring down Liver Yang.

There are so many ways to go wrong. You can misread the pulses and tongue; you can fail to gather crucial information, or fail to realise the importance of a piece of information you've been given; you can draw the wrong inference from what you see and hear; or you can, as I did, unaccountably overlook an obvious diagnosis. I could go on. The point is that we are all bound to get our diagnosis wrong sometimes, however diligent and careful and experienced we are. So what we need to learn is how to spot our mistakes as soon as possible. Then we need to learn how to correct them. But the first step is the vital one. Unless you realise you've made a mistake you'll never put it right.

So how do we learn? Most people learn to drive a car (I mean a car with manual gears – what they call stick-shift in the USA) even though it isn't easy. At first it is hard to find that point of balance between the left and right feet, between clutch and accelerator, which gets the car to start slowly and gather speed smoothly. People get the hang of it because they get instant and accurate feedback. The car stalls, or it leapfrogs down the road in a series of wild jumps, or the engine races and nothing happens. No possibility of doubt that you've got it wrong, and pretty clear exactly how you've got it wrong. There is, in short, a good feedback system.

So, in order to test our diagnoses, we need to create the same sort of thing in our own work. A feedback system boils down to the following. First, you need to know how the system should react (i.e. pull away smoothly); second you need to know how far it deviates from that (i.e. stalling or jumping) and lastly you need to know what to do to correct the error (i.e. let the clutch up more slowly).

Perhaps surprisingly, it is the first of these – How should the system react? – that is most often overlooked. It is crucial. This is the one you need to build into your way of working. For it generates the key question, the wonderful question, what, exactly, am I expecting from this treatment? And you can ask the same question of one treatment and of a series of treatments, whatever number you choose; what, exactly, am I expecting from these three, or six, or ten treatments?

To start with, take the question to refer to a single treatment. You might predict a particular pulse change, as discussed in the previous chapter, or a change in the patient's complaint, for example the easing of pain or the fading of a headache. But don't forget that this is energy medicine and that what you are doing, fundamentally, is bringing about a change in the patient's energy state. Of course there are some ailments that can't be treated by acupuncture, but for the rest we work on the basis that the patient's condition stems from his or her energy state and will improve if it changes.

So, to provide a baseline, how would you describe the patient's energy at the start of the session? Flat, tense, chaotic, weary, struggling, resigned? As soon as you've expressed any of these perceptions then it becomes obvious what change to expect. The opposites are: lifted, relaxed, organised, refreshed, calm, hopeful.

Some of these changes will be easier to spot than others. Relaxed or calm should be straightforward. Hopeful and lifted are harder. But, again, it isn't so difficult once you have the idea. For hopeful you might ask the patient about something he or she is facing in the following week and see if there is a shift in his or her attitude towards it. You might see it in the eyes; a change from passivity to a look of interest in, and engagement with, the world outside. As for lifted, you might notice that the patient's tone of voice has changed, that what was a flat monotone now has some variety, some lilt. You might also see a difference in the way he or she moves; if getting onto the couch was a slow weary business then you will be alert to notice if the patient gets off more quickly, and with more vigour.

You will also be predicting what will happen between this treatment and the next one. Naturally, if you are dealing with a chronic condition, especially in an elderly person, you might decide that one treatment won't make any real difference; but then you have to decide how many you do have to do before you can expect some change, otherwise you can find yourself persisting with a mistaken diagnosis for much longer than you should.

Another source of error comes from bad habits. They can grow up slowly over the years without our really noticing, especially as we start to develop our own style of working. I was taught, for example, not to treat at all at the first appointment but to spend well over an hour taking a very full case history and then to write up my notes before starting to treat at the second session. Well, I didn't like that. My first few patients arrived with quite severe conditions and it felt awful to simply talk to them and then turn them away without having done anything to help. So when I started to work on my own I decided that I would cut the talking a bit short in the first session and add a simple treatment. I made sure that I continued to take the case history over the next couple of sessions until it was complete; but as time went by I got sloppy and I ended up doing it only that first session, which meant that I was only taking about half the time over it that I had been taught was necessary. So I was probably not collecting important information, and therefore I was also reducing my chances of reaching an accurate diagnosis. Not a good habit.

It's hard to spot your own bad habits. In other parts of our lives we have friends and partners who very kindly point them out, usually more than once. But with your work there's no one to do that, so you have to do it for yourself.

One way of doing it is to jot down all the ways in which your practice deviates from what you were taught, and then consider the risks of that. It could be something as simple as where you have your sharps box (is it too far from the patient?); or it might be how carefully you record each treatment (do you put down pulse qualities?); or even how much trouble you take over your initial diagnosis (do you take the time to sketch out the connections between the patient's signs and symptoms and the diagnostic categories you use, and then revise and refine your first attempt?). If you're anything like me, you'll find there are some ways in which you have started to cut corners, to leave out the bits you find difficult or tedious, and they will be the source of mistakes.

The other basic way of identifying bad habits is to look through the records of those patients who are not doing as well as you'd hoped. The chances are that in at least some of these cases such habits have become crucial, so it is here that you are most likely to spot them. Take notes as you read. Which treatments worked well and which didn't?

Can you see any pattern? Did you use mainly command points, mainly points on the back or front of the body, mainly tonification, even or dispersal needle technique? Did you take fewer notes than usual? Then compare what you've noticed with the notes of a patient you've treated successfully. You'll see the difference.

Now for the business of correcting your errors. Imagine you've decided your diagnosis must be wrong in some way; you thought your patient would show signs of real improvement after three treatments, and she hasn't. The question is what to do about it. Sometimes, you just know. You look at her on the couch and you suddenly realise that Liver Qi stagnation needs to be dispersed, or that her constitutional element is Fire. But that doesn't often happen, and practitioners usually fiddle with the initial diagnosis, treating more syndromes or adding more pathogenic factors. The trouble with that is that it leads to treatments which become ever more complex, so it becomes ever harder to know what is really helping and what isn't. Better, I think, to go back to basics. Ask yourself, is this person's energy full or deficient? Is the problem one of Qi or Blood? Is there a block of some sort, which is preventing the treatment from working? Which element is in most distress? One of these questions, maybe all four, will yield a sensible treatment plan. Admittedly it will not amount to a full diagnosis of the kind you were taught in college, but it will get you out of a hole, and safely too. Plenty of time to come to a new diagnosis, as long as what you are doing in the meantime is helping and not making the patient worse.

The reason these questions will help is that they all point in the same direction, which is to ask you to look again at your patient's energy. Just now, reading this book, think of a patient whom you are finding difficult to treat, and imagine that he or she is sitting in front of you. Now, is that person's energy full or deficient? It may be immediately obvious; perhaps you are conjuring up someone with a pale white face, withdrawn, easily startled; or someone with quick movements who drops things, talks fast and rushes out of the room at the end of the session. That's pretty clear.

If you can't put your patient into either category then the source of her condition isn't so much to do with quantity of energy but quality. So try the question about the elements. You might remember, for example, that when she is quiet, perhaps as you take her pulses, there is an air of desolation about her, a profound sadness in her eyes. And then you remember that it all started with a bout of pneumonia ten years ago, and that she has had sinus problems ever since. A conviction comes over you to treat the lungs, starting with something simple like Bl 13 and Lu 9, maybe adding LI 4, but not straying outside the Metal element.

One last example. I treated a woman who had a mastectomy of her left breast because of a cancerous tumour there. After the operation she was in a lot of pain, had some lingering inflammation, and kept getting accumulations of fluid which had to be drained periodically. She was struggling emotionally, too, with the loss of a part of herself. I gave her a few treatments but they made no real difference. So I sat back and looked at her afresh. That's when I realised that she seemed frozen somehow, rigid, clenched. And I suddenly thought, 'She's still under anaesthetic.' So, for the first time, I asked permission to put my hands on her chest and feel what it was like. Same sort of thing. There was no life, no flow of energy through her chest area. I decided to needle Sp 21 and then Ht 1, and that released some sort of blockage in the area. After that she started to recover.

These examples all make the same point, which is that if your diagnosis isn't working the solution is to make it more simple not more complex. And, as a rule, that means getting out of your head, out of your thinking brain (for you can talk yourself into any and every diagnosis, and they'll all be equally plausible!). As a matter of fact, you can't work out what a person's energy is like; you have to perceive it. And, if you are anything like me, the fundamental reason why you aren't doing well with a particular patient is that you've forgotten to do that. You have got so tangled up with cause and effect, with syndromes and pathogens and point combinations and pulse qualities, with trying to make sense of divergent signs and inconsistent symptoms that you've lost sight of what you treat, which is the patient's energy. And to get back to that you need to tell your chattering mind, which has a hundred ideas a minute, to be quiet so you can open your senses to your patient.

Mistakes of technique, that is, the kind of mistakes you make in the course of a treatment, are usually quite easy to put right. I'm thinking of errors like needling the wrong point, mistaking Bl 60 for Ki 3 as I have done, or more forgivably, Bl 12 for 13 or Ki 24 for 25; or missing the point altogether; doing too many or too few points; using moxa when it doesn't suit the patient, and so on. (I don't include, here, the crucial error of tonifying when you should be dispersing, or vice versa, because this is really an error of diagnosis.)

This is where taking pulses throughout the treatment can really help. You needle a point and take the pulses. Crudely, there are three possible responses. First, they improve, which means that you got the point and it was a good choice. Second, there is no change in the pulses, so either you missed the point (try again), or it was irrelevant (in which case don't bother). Finally, if the pulses get worse, then you got the point but it wasn't what the patient needed. So you have to rethink.

There is a lovely twist to this which I have seen more often than I care to admit. I needle the wrong point and before I correct myself I take the pulses, just to see what's happened, and the result is terrific. In fact, it's a better pulse change than I was expecting from the point I'd chosen. Wonderful. I feel so grateful when this happens because it means I've been led to what the patient needs in spite of myself and in spite of my failings as a practitioner. It also gives me an enormous clue as to what's wrong with my diagnosis. In fact, I sometimes wonder if I am being led, unconsciously, away from what I intended and towards what is actually the best point for that patient, it certainly feels like that sometimes. So don't be in too much of a hurry to correct a mistake, for it just may be one of those rare but precious gifts.

There is one other category of mistakes and that is mistakes in managing the process of treatment. After all, taking on a new patient is the start of a relationship which may last months or even years, and the relationship will need to be maintained and deepened if you are to do the best for him or her. This is a big topic so I will consider it separately in the next chapter.

Finally, there is the question of whether or not to admit your mistakes. When I was a student, the most senior teacher at the college was adamant that you should never tell a patient that you had made a mistake. I thought he was wrong then and I think he's wrong now. You will have to come to your own conclusion about this, but do consider your own attitude to this issue because it will influence the nature of your relationship with your patients.

For me, it starts with the simplest thing, which is missing a point. I do it all the time. As I bend over the patient, to needle again in nearly the same place as before, it seems natural to say that I missed the point the first time and want to have another try. I don't apologise (or not usually, and even then not cravenly). That would suggest to the patient that I shouldn't ever miss a point, that I am incompetent for having done so, and that I may have done some sort of harm by missing it. None of which is true.

Some practitioners don't say they've missed the point. They just don't say anything at all. This rather assumes that the patient is passive, won't wonder why they are being needled again in almost exactly the same place and that he or she just takes it for granted that you are doing the right thing. That may be true for many patients, but notice the effect it will have on the relationship, and perhaps on the atmosphere in the treatment room too. It will tend to make patients see you as an expert, as someone working with technical and arcane knowledge which they cannot possibly understand, in much the same way, perhaps, as they see their doctor. They are given the medicine, so to speak, and they take it. In this way of working, feedback tends to be limited. Patients may tell their doctor if the prescribed medicine has really unpleasant side effects, but otherwise most people assume it must be doing them good and carry on taking it, even if there is not much evidence that it is; indeed, often in the teeth of evidence that it isn't. The expert knows best.

It may suit you to work in this way, and it is certainly true that there are patients who do not want their practitioner to talk about the treatments or to explain what he or she is doing and why. I suppose it follows that they don't want to know about errors either. I have patients like this, but I am conscious that I find it a bit of a strain working with them. It goes against my natural inclination, so I am probably not the best practitioner for them.

That's normal. We each have our own style of working and few of us are comfortable with every single one of our patients. My bias is to engage the patient as fully as possible in the course of treatment, so naturally I talk about what I am doing and why, and equally naturally some patients find it tedious or aggravating. One of them once said, charmingly, 'If it's all the same to you, I came for a treatment not a lecture.' Fair enough. On the other hand, I recently treated a young woman in her twenties whose periods became agonisingly painful about 18 months ago. She loved the lecture. Before that, she explained, the pain had seemed like some kind of random cruelty inflicted on her by a capricious body, and she could see no prospect of change. Once she understood the cause of the pain, which included why it had started just then, she could see how and why it might stop. That made a huge difference.

In the end, the message of this chapter, as indeed of all the others, is to find a way of working that suits you, which satisfies that part of you which wanted to become an acupuncturist in the first place and which leaves you at the end of a long day in the treatment room still feeling passionate about your work. And your way of dealing with your mistakes will be an important aspect of this. If they get to you and sap your confidence they will gradually erode your joy in the work, and indeed your effectiveness. If, on the other hand, you can find a way of integrating them into your vision of what you are doing and why – well, you may still wince at some of the things you've done, but you will make creative use of them and treat them as a ladder to higher levels of skill.

CHAPTER 6

PATIENTS

Some years ago, when I moved to a new part of the country and had to wind up my acupuncture practice, I thought it would be interesting to look through my records and analyse what had happened to my patients. In particular, I wanted to see if there were any clues as to why some people got better and some did not. I thought it would be helpful to know if, for example, I hadn't done well with irritable bowel syndrome or migraines, or with people who came because their husband or wife wanted them to come; and I wanted to find out if I'd been successful with certain conditions like depression or asthma or with certain types of patients, such as those who had already tried Western medicine. With that information I thought I'd be able to give better information to prospective patients.

I tried all the obvious criteria. I looked to see if young people were more likely to get better than old ones; if recent acute problems and injuries cleared up more easily than chronic ones; if success depended on how enthusiastic, or how sceptical, the patient was about his treatment, and so on. None of these criteria worked. For example, I saw a woman in her fifties who had had a major restriction in her shoulder since she was a little girl, and it cleared with one treatment. On the other hand, I saw a young man who had cricked his neck on a flight back from America only a couple of weeks earlier, and after three treatments there was no improvement whatsoever. It was the same story wherever I looked. An old Irish man who came into the clinic announcing loudly, 'I don't believe in all this new age nonsense you know,' got enormous help with his chronic diabetes, while I made absolutely no difference to the minor stomach complaint of a woman who was passionately enthusiastic about complementary medicine.

Eventually I found two criteria which made sense. The first was relatively easy to spot (the second took me years). It was to do with how well patients reported on the effect of each treatment. It wasn't so much that most of the patients who got better had given me good feedback, though that was the case. Much more important was the finding that virtually none of the other patients, the ones who didn't get better, had given me good feedback.

I am sure this is no coincidence. I would ask, 'How have you been this week?' and the answer would come back, 'Fine,' or 'Pretty bad,' or 'Much the same.' I would go on, 'So, did you still feel cold in bed, like last week?' Or perhaps, 'Did you manage to move your bowels each day?' and the answer would always be vague; they weren't sure, they thought it might have been a bit better, they couldn't remember and so on – in spite of the fact that I had explained the importance of keeping some sort of brief record so that we would know whether or not the treatment was working.

It's not surprising, once you think about it, that I failed with these patients. For one thing, without feedback I didn't know if my diagnosis was brilliant, alright or just plain wrong. How could I tell? So there was no opportunity to change a wrong diagnosis or refine an mediocre one. What was even worse, in a funny sort of a way, was wondering if my diagnosis had been spot on first time (highly unusual I admit). That's because the vague feedback made me lose faith in it and try something else, taking the patient's diffidence as a sign that I wasn't on the right track.

There's another aspect to this as well, which I can best explain by contrasting inadequate feedback with that produced by a patient who, each week, gave me a drawing of her back. Areas of pain were marked on the drawing, and the markings were darker or lighter to show how acute the pain had been. On that basis we could look together at why one week might have been better than another, or why the pain might have shifted location. I tried a few different kinds of treatment to see which worked best for her, and got a clear answer. We also discovered that the week she had to drive her car more than usual was an especially bad week, and that led to a change in her car seat which made a huge difference.

Unlike the patients who didn't give me any real feedback, she was participating in her recovery. She didn't expect me to simply fix her back without her doing anything, changing anything. She took responsibility for finding out what helped and what didn't, and then took responsibility for doing everything she could to do more of the first and less of the second. That changed everything. Not least, it removed a tremendous burden from my shoulders. I didn't have to do it all, and I didn't have to do it alone, and that in itself seemed to free me up to work with more conviction and more power.

On the patient's side, I think it marks an important psychological shift. Taking time and trouble each day to record the progress of treatment, even if it only takes a minute, shows a willingness to do what it takes to get better. Some people, though they may not be aware of it, lack this. They may feel defeated by their illness; they may have given up hope in some deep way; or they may be lazy and prefer, actually, to stay as they are rather than make a serious effort to improve; they may not realise that they have built their lives around being unwell, and the prospect of getting better may be alarming, frightening even. Unconsciously, they may consider that while life may not be all that good as it is, perhaps it would be worse if everything were to change. I do not mean to blame these patients. They have not deliberately chosen these attitudes; it's more that they have grown up over the years as a result of their experiences, usually painful ones at that. The point is that beliefs of this kind form a real barrier to treatment, and one simple way to try and loosen the hold they have is to get the patient to take good notes of the effects of each treatment.

If you have patients who do not give you good feedback and who also seem stuck, then I think that persuading them to take good notes between sessions may be the most important thing you can do to make treatment more effective.

Although this issue was important I knew there was more to discover about my practice. What was the difference between those patients who got better and those who did not? As is often the way when you can't find an answer to a question, it's because it was the wrong question. There was no difference between the patients. The difference was in me.

For example, I have a patient who drives me crazy. I have treated her, on and off, for about ten years. 'Off,' because sometimes I have pushed her away, told her there's no more I can do for her, or sent her to other practitioners. But she always comes back. She sits there, listing an endless series of tiny, minor complaints, most of which can't be treated with acupuncture, while I fret about having not enough time to treat her or running late for the rest of the day. Then, as she's leaving the room at the end of her treatment and I'm putting away her notes and beginning to gear myself up for the next person, she stops with her hand on the door knob and says, 'Oh there's one thing I forgot to tell you about...' or 'There's something I'd like to ask you...' It makes me want to run screaming from the room, tearing my hair. An excessive response, you might think, and you'd be right. What is it about her? Nothing. The question is, what is it about me?

Many years ago now I was given the most wonderful lesson by one of my teachers. I was in a class, working with a fellow student, trying to do what we had just been taught, which was how to evaluate the movements of the neck. I was finding it difficult. I wasn't holding her head confidently; I thought that my fingers were pulling on her hair, and worst of all I wasn't even learning anything because she was bracing her muscles and keeping hold of her head instead of letting me move it through its natural range of motion. I was struggling, not knowing how to do the work or how to deal with the situation. Just then I glanced up and saw that the teacher was watching me. I felt so embarrassed, so stupid and incompetent. And, I am ashamed to say, I didn't want him to think that, so I turned to him and said, 'She won't let me take her head; she keeps hanging on to it.' He smiled in a kindly way, 'No,' he said. 'You're not holding her head in such a way that she feels able to relax.'

Exactly. That's the truth. Don't blame the patient. It was my job as a practitioner to find a way to make her comfortable with whatever had to be done to make the treatment effective and help the process of healing. Just as it is your job with your patients. And some of them will be difficult for you, just as the two I have mentioned were, in different ways, difficult for me.

And that's why I could find no criterion which distinguished those patients who got better from those who did not. It's because I was looking at the patients, and asking myself what they or their complaints had in common, when I should have been looking at myself. The patients who didn't get better were the ones I wasn't coping with, the ones whose heads, so to speak, I wasn't able to hold properly.

It sounds so simple on the page, but I assure you it was a revelation. I practically heard the thunder and saw the clouds parting and a bolt of lightening emerging and hitting me on the forehead.

Suddenly I could see how it was true of every single one of the patients who didn't get better. And then I realised that there were two ways in which I failed. Two ways which, I suspect, apply to all of us.

First were those patients I really, really wanted to get better. Of course I want all my patients to get better, but I have to admit that there is a spectrum, and with some of them my desire is strong. Perhaps I am particularly fond of them or feel especial sympathy for their plight; less forgivably, they are at the centre of a social network and I know that if they do well they will send me lots of other patients; perhaps they are famous and I am a sucker for famous people. Whatever, it is the very strength of my wish which gets in the way of treatment. I'll explain why in a moment, but first I'll describe the other category of patients.

This is composed of people who don't really interest me. It is a bit shocking to admit it, but I do find some of my patients boring. They tell me interminable stories about what has been going on in their lives, with excessive detail which has nothing to do with their complaint or their treatment, and I sit there rapidly losing interest. Others are patients for whom I have worked hard, trying everything I know, and who report no improvement. I can cope with that. What I find difficult is that after I have suggested that they try other therapies, or other practitioners, they insist on coming back. I ought to be pleased, flattered even, but I'm not, I'm bored. I can't get interested when I have nothing more to say or to do. And finally, there are some patients who come for a few treatments and, just as they are starting to get better, stop coming for a year or two – and then return with the same complaint. I lose interest after a few cycles like this because I know that as soon as there is a chance of really making a difference they will disappear again.

It may seem strange that the two categories are composed of opposites: people who bore me and those in whom I have an especial interest, but that is the clue to what is going on. I don't really see either of them clearly. What gets in the way, in both cases, are my own needs and interests. In both cases I am busy with something going on in my own head rather than simply paying attention to the patient.

The best practitioners have this particular ability, this great gift. They pay real attention to each patient. I quoted earlier the story of Yeshi Dhonden taking pulses, told by a doctor; here is a extract from the same piece, edited a little differently.

The patient had been awakened early and told that she is to be examined by a foreign doctor... She has long ago taken on that mixture of compliance and resignation that is the face of chronic illness... Yeshi Dhonden steps to the bedside while the rest of us stand apart, watching. For a long time he gazes at the women, favouring no part of her body with his eyes, but seeming to fix his glance at a place just above her supine form. I, too, study her. No physical sign or obvious symptom gives a clue as to the nature of her disease.

At last he takes her hand, raising it in both his own. Now he bends over the bed in a kind of crouching stance, his head drawn down into the collar of his robe. His eyes are closed as he feels for her pulse. In a moment he has found the spot, and for the next half-hour he remains thus…holding the pulse of the woman beneath his fingers… After a moment the woman rests back on her pillow. From time to time she raises her head to look at the strange figure above her, then sinks back once more… All at once I am envious – not of him, not of Yeshi Dhonden…but of her. I want to be held like that, touched so, *received*… At last Yeshi Dhonden straightens, gently places the woman's hand on the bed and steps back… All this while he has not uttered a single word.

As he nears the door, the woman raises her head and calls to him in a voice at once urgent and serene. 'Thank you, doctor,' she says, and touched with her other hand the place he had held on her wrist, as though to recapture something that had visited there. (Dass and Gorman 1992, pp.119–120)

Quite apart from the power of that thank you and all it implies, you might like to know how the story ends. This woman had undergone about 90 tests over a two-year period in one of the top hospitals in America before her doctors managed to arrive at the correct diagnosis. Yeshi Dhonden got it in that half-hour.

We can't all be as good as Yeshi Dhonden, but we can learn from him. And what we can learn is the power of simple attention. Not only did it give him the correct diagnosis, it made the patient feel better too.

I call this kind of attention 'simple' not to belittle it, but to describe it as pure, uncontaminated, absolute. If I am worrying too much about my patient, perhaps wanting to add a point to make the treatment especially good, or being particularly sympathetic, or making sure that I handle a limb extra gently, then I won't be paying simple attention; I'll be doing something with the specific intention of making the patient feel better. And I can't do two things at once. If I am working with an intention I can't, at the same time, be paying attention to the patient. The intention itself narrows the gaze, selects what is noticed, makes information fit into a predetermined pattern. But, as the story of Yeshi Dhonden suggests, it is simply by paying attention to our patients that we help them the most, because it leads us to the best diagnosis. And it is not determined efforts to help nor effusive sympathy which comforts the patient but simple attention. It provides such deep reassurance that even onlookers, like the doctor who told the story, feel envious.

This is a difficult thing to communicate in a society and in a culture which emphasises goals and achievement and effort. We are taught that it is by planning, by organising, by decision-making that we can make things happen and bring about change. In medicine, drugs are prescribed to kill specific bacteria, to reduce blood pressure, to disperse cholesterol; surgery removes diseased tissue, or reconstructs a worn joint. It is all intentional. There is no room for simple attention. It is even difficult to talk about it in our language. We have many verbs for particular ways of thinking; we analyse, reason, deliberate, weigh up, assess, judge, and so on, but there is no equivalent for paying attention. So the writer Robert Heinlen invented the verb 'grok'. Grokking is not the same as thinking; it is what happens when we really pay attention. It is a mixture of perceiving, intuiting, seeing, recognising and grasping all of something, all at once.

And that is what we need to try to do with our patients. We don't so much need to analyse them, work them out, or fit them into categories; we need to see them all at once, exactly as they are, just as Yeshi Dhonden did. Then we'll know how to help.

Finally I want to look at the issue of managing the process of treatment. After all, taking on a new patient is the start of a relationship which may last months or even years, and the relationship will need to be maintained and deepened if you are to do the best for him or her.

Most obviously, if a patient doesn't like the way you are with her, finding you too laid back, too bossy, too indecisive, whatever, then she might not come back. That might also happen if you treat friends, or become friends with those you treat, for if the friendship breaks down it will be hard to maintain the therapeutic relationship. No doubt these basics were taught and discussed as part of any acupuncture training, so here I will confine myself to a few core issues which turn up again and again in different guises until you have dealt with your own attitudes to them.

The first is any struggle for control. For example, if the patient comes for treatment at intervals which you do not recommend, but which he chooses; if he complains that you do not do the kinds of treatments which his previous practitioner did; if he is regularly late for treatment; if he pays you more, or less, than your fee; if he routinely rejects your advice – an especially important instance of this is if you insist that he doesn't have other forms of treatment for a while so you can get clear feedback on your work, but he carries on doing so. In all these cases you will need to assert yourself if the process is to work. When you treat someone you are making a serious intervention in his or her body, mind and spirit, and you cannot do it well, or safely, on terms dictated by someone who has no proper knowledge or understanding of that intervention. You simply cannot take responsibility for your work under these conditions, and if you can't take responsibility for it, perhaps you shouldn't be doing it in the first place.

The second issue is confusion about money. Any patient can turn up one day thinking she had her purse or her cheque book with her and finding she didn't. What matters is what happens next. If she pays without any fuss, either the next day or at the next treatment, well and good. But if she forgets again, or forgets regularly, then, probably unconsciously, she doesn't think the treatments are worth paying for.

The only way to deal with this, as with all these issues, is to turn your attention from the patient onto yourself. Instead of asking why she is mean or manipulative or forgetful, ask what you are doing that leads her to behave in this way. Have you suddenly lost confidence in what you are doing, either with her or more generally? Do you feel, deep down, that you have done all you can for her and you don't actually expect any more improvement? Has treatment got her through the initial crisis which brought her to you and neither of you quite knows what you are supposed to be doing now? Any of these feelings in you would go a long way to explaining her forgetfulness.

It may also have to do with your own attitude towards money and towards charging people for treatment. Few of us have a simple uncomplicated relationship with money, and it may be that this particular patient has sensed some ambivalence in you about your fee. Perhaps, for some reason, you would really prefer not to charge her at all; or you wish that you had some sort of a sliding scale of charges so you could ask less from her and more from some of your wealthier patients. The variety is huge; the point is that if you find that patients are forgetting to pay, or finding your arrangements for payment complicated or difficult, the chances are that you have some unresolved issues with money which you will need to sort out so they don't get in the way of the process of treatment.

Finally, there is the frustration of those patients who will not do anything to help themselves. Earlier in this chapter I discussed how vital it is that they do so; here I want to look what you might be doing which, somehow or other, gives the patient permission to behave as they do. If most of your patients fail to cooperate then you are probably lacking confidence in yourself and in your right to insist that they participate in their own recovery. What is it that you doubt? What would help you to banish that doubt?

More likely it is one or two patients who habitually ignore your advice and suggestions, so the issue is to do with your specific attitudes to them. Speaking personally, there are two types of patients with whom I know I fail in this way. One is men who have prestigious jobs and are, in consequence, much richer than I am. Some of them are famous too. Although I know it is stupid of me, I do hesitate to tell them what to do. There is probably some deep psychological explanation – perhaps I see them as I saw my father when I was a small child – and I would certainly never have dared tell him what to do. The other type is attractive women who are having a hard time in life. Instinctively I want to carry their burden rather than adding to it by giving them tasks to do, especially if they are difficult ones. No doubt the kind of patients who catch you out will be different, but I'd be surprised if you don't have any with whom you're a bit reluctant to be firm.

You'll be pleased to hear that there is no need to plumb the depths of your psyche in order to sort this out. Knowing your weakness is almost enough in itself. For my part, now when I find myself hesitating to ask, 'So did you manage to go for a walk every day last week?' or, 'Did you stop work when you felt tired, or did you carry on as usual?' I can smile at myself, recognising the old pattern. And then

I can make a sort of accommodation. It wouldn't be right to let the patient off the hook completely, for it wouldn't be in his or her best interests. But nor do I have to force myself to do something I find hard; not least because I may then end up not doing it at all. So the compromise is something like, 'Tell me you walked once this week!' That lightens it a bit, possibly for both of us. Or, feeling I need to be serious rather than jovial, I might say, 'I can pick you back up again with this treatment, back to where you were last week, but you won't move forward until you can cut down on work.'

When I think of the best practitioners I have had the privilege of knowing, I notice one thing that they have in common and which distinguishes them from their colleagues. It is that they can treat whoever comes through the door, the arrogant and the timid, the wise and the foolish, the chronically ill and the hypochondriac. They seem to be able to see through whatever front the patient puts on and recognise the person beneath, the one who has always been there. I have a photograph of my father, aged about eight, and in the photo he has a look in his eye which I saw in him at the age of 99, shortly before he died. It is who he was. And the best practitioners would have seen that, and treated it.

In the first few years of practice you will get good results with those patients you can see clearly, probably ones who are like you in some important way and who aren't challenging. They don't, as the phrase has it, push your buttons. You don't react to them by being especially diligent, or anxious, or careful, or compliant, or impatient, or sympathetic, or anything. Then, as time goes by, you will find that you are treating people with whom you have really nothing in common and getting good results. What seems to happen then is that patients start to turn up who you find difficult; it is almost as if someone has noticed that it is time for you to extend your range, to overcome your limitations as a practitioner, and has sent you a carefully selected bunch of awkward customers. When it happens, you will be tested. You will find yourself being manipulated, losing confidence and getting stressed. It is normal; it is just a sign that you are now taking on a wider range of patients and conditions and that you are outside your comfort zone. Hang on. And remember that the way through is to let go of wanting those patients to be more friendly, more interesting, more appreciative, whatever it is that you love about the others, and just see them for who they really are. Then you'll find them easy.

CHAPTER 7

SUCCESS AND FAILURE

In the early days of practice it seems so straightforward. Success is when the patient gets better and failure is when he or she does not. And sometimes it really is like that. I recently treated a young woman who, for the last couple of years, has had very bad period pains and after only two treatments she was astonished and delighted to have a painless period. Simple. But most of the time it really isn't as simple as that. In fact, for reasons I'll explain later, even my young woman's case turned out to be a bit more complicated than it seemed.

In the early days of practice people tend to come to you for pretty obvious reasons: to deal with pain, to alleviate some condition like migraines or asthma or constipation, to help them break an addiction to cigarettes or alcohol, or to lose weight. But as you get more experienced you'll find yourself treating a wider range of patients and a wider range of conditions, and that will raise the issue of how best to assess your treatments.

One of the first times this happened to me was when I treated an elderly woman for tinnitus. The treatment worked reasonably well, though not perfectly, and she asked me if I expected any further improvement. I said I thought not, and she was interested. How come, she wanted to know, acupuncture could make her tinnitus a lot better but not completely better? A good question, and in the course of my answer I touched on some fundamental issues to do with health and healing and concluded by saying that although acupuncture could have a profound effect on some illnesses and disease states, I saw it more as preventive medicine, more as a way of maintaining and amplifying health. 'Oh,' she said, 'if I chose to come to you to maintain my health, how often would I have to come?' As she was in her mid sixties at the time I replied, 'About once a month.' And she and her husband have come once a month ever since, even though I have moved away from where they live and they have to travel over an hour to see me.

This couple has taught me such a lot over the years, and one of the great lessons is that I couldn't use my usual criteria to decide if my treatments were working. Would they have stayed well without treatment? No way of knowing. When they did fall ill, could I have prevented it if my treatments had been better? Again, no way of knowing. So how could I tell if I needed to change my diagnosis or use different treatment techniques? How could I tell if I was doing a good job or not?

A more extreme example of the same issue is when you come to treat people who are terminally ill. You know that you are not going to make them better so you have to find some other way of thinking about what you are doing and how well you are doing it. And then you can take what you learn from that experience back into your more usual work.

One more instance. A middle-aged man came for treatment because he was overweight; not a tall man, he weighed nearly 18 stone, had high blood pressure and a good deal of anxiety. He was trapped in the kind of vicious circle familiar to those with any kind of addiction; he knew that he smoked too many cigarettes and drank too much alcohol, and he felt bad about it, so he would smoke and drink some more in order to comfort himself. Over the course of a year of treatment he didn't lose much weight, but all sorts of other things changed. For one thing, his body shape altered quite dramatically. He lost his protruding belly and seemed to put more weight onto his upper body, broadening his shoulders. That made him feel better. He also discovered a source of hidden grief and resentment about the way his father had treated him and he began to appreciate the fact that he had needed to find a way to cope with it, and he realised that cigarettes and alcohol had become his way. As a result of all that, he started to feel he hadn't done so badly after all, in the circumstances. And because of that insight he started to take better care of himself and he cut down on his addictions very substantially. The process is still going on. We both think that treatment has been successful, but if we had judged it on the simple criterion of whether or not he has lost any significant amount of weight, we'd have decided it was a failure. Here is a conversation between patient and practitioner which sums up the issue very neatly.

At the end of a series of sessions I try to get feedback
from my clients. I need to know what is working for
people and what isn't. One of the first times I did this
was with a powerful woman lawyer. During the last
session I said to her very formally that I thought it
would be a good idea to review what had happened
here.

'That would be wonderful,' she said.

'Grand,' I said. 'I'd like to ask you, did you get
what you came for?'

She replied 'Absolutely not.'

I was flabbergasted. I asked her what she meant.

She said, 'Rachel, when I came here I didn't know
that what I got even existed.' (Ramen 1989, p.93)

That's a wonderful tribute both to the practitioner and to
this system of medicine, showing how it offers far more
than the relief of whatever symptoms the patient brings
to you at that first session. But unless you have a patient
as aware and as eloquent as Rachel's it can be difficult to
judge whether or not you are doing good work.

It is so important to be realistic in your judgements.
There's a real danger in feeling you've failed if your patient
doesn't get better, and probably an even greater danger in
claiming a success every time one of your patients does
well. The fact is quite a few of your patients won't get
better – ask any practitioner who has been doing this work
for a long time and they'll tell you it's true. So the question
is, how do you deal with that? If you feel responsible,
believing that if only you had been able to come to the

right diagnosis, or the right point combination, or seen them more often, or hit all the points (it doesn't matter what you pick as the cause of the failure) then I don't think you will enjoy the work and I do think you will get exhausted and feel defeated by it. That's too heavy a burden to carry, especially when you are busy and have many patients who are seriously unwell, and you will worry, burn out, get depressed, whichever way you tend to crack under pressure.

I'm not saying you should ignore the effect of your treatments on your patients, still less that you shouldn't learn from your mistakes. What I am saying is that you should do your best, working carefully and conscientiously, taking time and trouble in the treatment room and being forever open to learning; but that's the extent of your responsibility. You cannot take responsibility for the outcome of treatment. Apart from the consequences for your own well-being, which I've mentioned, there's a more fundamental reason why it is wrong to do so; which is that you are not in control of your patient's body or healing.

For one thing, however frequently you treat him or her, it is still a tiny amount of time in relation to the rest of that patient's life, and what happens outside the treatment room will be just as important, probably more important, than what you do. If your patient is in a loving family which supports and encourages her path back to health and has a sympathetic employer in a job she loves, you can be sure that the prognosis will be better than if she lives alone and hates her job.

More fundamentally, acupuncture, like every other system of medicine, doesn't cure people or heal them; only nature can do that.

Think of something simple like a cut on the ball of your thumb. You can create conditions which will help it to heal, putting on antiseptic cream to prevent infection, covering it with a plaster to keep it clean, maybe stitching it up if the cut is deep, but you can't heal it. That's a natural process far more sophisticated and far more powerful than any medicine. And if that's true for a cut, it must be true for the more complex conditions which you treat every day.

So if your patient didn't get better there are a thousand possible reasons why that was so, and you will almost certainly never know why. It is genuinely helpful to accept that for all the brilliance and wisdom of acupuncture, for all its history of thousands of years of successful practice and clinical experience, for all the knowledge you have accumulated at college and since, nevertheless you are dealing all day and every day with something which ultimately remains a mystery. Given the brilliance of the theories, concepts and techniques of acupuncture, we don't really know how it works. Incidentally, the same is true of most modern medicine. Drugs don't always work on everyone as theory predicts, and, of course, every surgeon relies on the body's own healing to carry on the process which he or she has initiated, not least by binding up the flesh which has been cut open.

You might think you're being modest if you say that you should have made some patient better. In fact, it's more likely that you are being arrogant. Blaming yourself for failure rests on the same underlying assumption as taking credit for success; that you have the power to heal someone. Both are untrue. If you take credit for successes, and you have a lot of them, then you may not get exhausted and burnt out, but you may become conceited and end up with an uncomfortably large ego.

I seem to be putting forward a very strange argument. First that it isn't easy to assess what you do, and second that you shouldn't get too involved in whether or not it works. I agree that it doesn't sound right, but so far all I have done is point out the problems of a simple attitude to success or failure; for the rest of the chapter I'll explain how you can in fact tell if your work is a success or not, and I'll explain how it is possible to care deeply for your patients without taking on the role of saviour or healer.

There are a few basic ways you can tell if you are doing a good job. One is simply by looking back over your notes. If you have a patient who isn't doing well, or about whom you are unsure in some way, then review the treatments you've done and notice your reaction. If you say to yourself, 'Yes, those are nice treatments,' or, 'I can see how I followed that diagnosis clearly and thoroughly,' or, 'That makes sense,' then I think you can rest assured that you've done as well as you could – and after all, what more can you do? If, on the other hand, you find yourself saying things like, 'Hmm, that treatment is a bit all over the place,' or, 'I don't quite know what I was getting at there,' or, 'I seem to have been chopping and changing a lot' (all examples from my own experience!), then you know you've lost your way.

Next, if you are in any doubt as to whether or not you are helping, it's a good idea to express to yourself, in a few words, what your patient really wants from treatment. Some of them aren't coming, in fact, for the relief of symptoms. For example, I have two patients who are different in almost every way but they both come to me for support. One is a middle-aged woman married to a very successful public figure. What she needs is somewhere to go, once a month, where she can speak without having to mind her words and where someone will listen to her without judging her. The needles relax her and relieve a bit of the tension she holds, but they aren't what really helps. The other patient is a young female shamanic healer. She is good at what she does but doubts her calling. What she gets from the experience of being treated herself is a reminder that this is indeed her work, that she is acutely sensitive to the flows of energy in her body, and that she is unusual in this respect. I sum that up, as with the first patient, as needing support. So I know that the right question to ask about their treatments is simply, 'Am I giving these patients the support they need?'

Another way of assessing your work, probably the one you'll use the most, comes through observing changes to basic functions like sleep, digestion, bowel movements, breathing, menstruation and so on. Offhand, I can't think of a single example of a patient who, along with his or her main complaint, hasn't had problems with at least one of these functions. I treat a woman who came for treatment because her hair was falling out; she also had irregular periods. Similarly, I see many people with asthma or persistent bronchitis and they are often also chronically constipated. It's pretty clear why it is so common. In general, it's because a weakness in one function is bound to have an effect on others. But in this specific example it's probably because as the breath comes in, the diaphragm should move down and press onto the organs that lie beneath it, and the large intestine lies directly beneath the diaphragm. So if a patient's breathing is shallow and high in the chest, then the large intestine isn't being massaged regularly, and without that massage it is harder for it to move its contents.

Just as a limitation in one function will hinder some other one, it follows that an improvement in one will help the others. A patient has come because of a skin complaint, acne, eczema or rashes, and after a few treatments there is no sign that they are clearing up. Carry on with the treatment or not? A good test is to see if there is any improvement in his basic systems. Is his constipation better? His sleep? His headaches? His general tiredness? If so, then I would reckon that the treatment is working, it just hasn't done enough yet to reach the skin, or to reverse what must have been a long disease process, but the chances are it will.

Along the same lines, what often happens after a few treatments is that a patient will say there isn't much improvement in his original complaint but that he has more energy. That is definitely a good sign. If muscles and ligaments, organs and blood are not working as well and efficiently as they should, then it takes a lot of energy to keep them functioning well enough to keep the body viable.

The same is true of emotions. The natural flow of the energy of anger, for example, is to come up from the liver and outwards. If, for some reason, a person cannot allow this anger to flow along its natural course, then it must be held in, and it takes an enormous amount of energy to do so, energy which must have been diverted from enabling some other function. You can sometimes see the effect of holding this energy in. It tends to produce a stiffness in the area of the diaphragm which then throws the chest outwards, pushes the shoulders back and the neck forward. So, if treatment is helping the patient's body, mind and spirit to work more easily then the energy that has been released, and which the patient tells you about, will be available for other things, and in particular it will be available for healing.

In a normal day, going to bed tired, we will have used up more or less all of our energy. So it makes sense that if we have to do something extra, such as recovering from the flu, mending a broken limb or getting over an operation, then we need to make sure we have enough for the job, and acupuncture treatments which release energy currently being used up unnecessarily is a good way to do it. Therefore, when your patient says that he has more energy you can be confident that your treatment is working, and you may need to remind him not to use it up on doing more, because it will be needed for healing.

The overall effect of acupuncture on a person's energy levels explains another reaction to treatment, one which you need to notice when you have patients with deep-seated chronic, or even terminal, conditions. When you are treating patients like this it is easy to become disheartened. Week after week there seems to be no improvement, and indeed often their condition will get worse, and you are bound to wonder if you are doing anything at all to help, and whether it would be more honest to stop. I have been in this position many times and always find it difficult. But I have found one good test which helps.

The starting point is to realise that there can be a difference between pain and suffering. I have a patient who was crippled in an industrial accident and will now spend the rest of his life in a wheelchair, and everyone who comes into his presence feels inspired, uplifted, joyous. He is often in pain but he relishes his life, and it makes sense to say that he isn't suffering. Or, to take a more normal example, practically everyone has had their heart broken at one time or another, when a loved one dies or a relationship ends, and it is very distressing. But whereas most of us get over it, there are some who never really recover, and even when they are no longer in pain their suffering comes to dominate their lives. The point is that with some of your patients you may not be able to do anything to relieve their pain, physical or emotional, but you may very well be helping to assuage their suffering.

To some extent this will come simply from your presence, from your willingness to turn up week after week (I have more to say about this later in the book). But there is one specific way of telling if your treatments are helping and that is when you notice a shift of energy in the room. It's quite hard to describe this, though once you've been alerted to the possibility and been assured that it is a genuine phenomenon, it isn't hard to spot. There are a number of signs. One is that the air seems lighter, brighter, clearer. Another that it is as if something has been holding its breath for a long time and has suddenly relaxed with an out breath. Occasionally, the walls seem to back away, giving you and your patient more space. Usually, there is an atmosphere of calm and quiet, almost of certainty.

Explanations of this phenomenon differ but there is no doubt that it is real. Given that we are talking about energy medicine here, let me suggest that what has happened is that treatment has brought about a profound change in the patient's energy state, a change that may not be strong enough to make a difference to a chronic condition or an advanced disease but which is certainly strong enough to bring her some peace and calm in the face of it, and hence relieve some of her suffering. And because it is such a profound shift it is not confined to the patient's body but spills out into the room. You can't help but notice it, for it will affect you as it affects everything else around. And actually, you can't help but relish it, for it is a rare and wonderful sensation. And it tells you, unmistakably, that your treatments are working well.

Which brings me back to the conversation I quoted earlier in this chapter when a patient told her practitioner that 'When I came here I didn't know that what I got even existed.' The tests I have mentioned do not judge the success of a treatment or course of treatments according to changes in the patient's initial symptoms, for the very good reason that the most important changes are often the ones the patient didn't come for, didn't expect, and could not have imagined. Most people who come for treatment assume that the best they can hope for is that they will be restored to the state they were in before they became ill or unwell, before some system failed or became compromised. But acupuncture can do more, and do better, than that.

For one thing, a lot of the patients you will see have been living in a way that practically guarantees problems; they eat poor food on the run; they don't get enough sleep; they wear shoes which put a terrible strain on their knees and hips; they put up with a job they hate or a relationship that doesn't nourish them; they carry on working when they aren't feeling well, thereby lowing their resistance to illness. For them, getting back to normal is not enough. One of the profound effects of treatment for such patients is that they start to feel really well for the first time for years, and that encourages them to make changes in their life so that they can keep it up. In fact, one criterion of success is really an educational one; whether or not your patients learn to take better care of themselves.

And at a deeper level, treatment can help people realise their full potential. There are patients who, when you are sitting opposite them, suddenly seem to you as if they should really be bigger, more powerful, more capable, more talented than they appear, and usually than they have come to believe. It is as if they have turned down the volume of their true character or personality, have pulled back a little into the shadows, have shrunk a little in the wash of life. If, as I have suggested, acupuncture can release all the energy which was previously used to prop up a struggling system, then that energy becomes available for living life to the full. Some of your patients may have given up on who they would like to be and what they would like to do because the challenge of daily life takes up all their energy and they don't have any left over for following their dreams. If treatment can give them more energy, or organise their energy better so it can do more work, then all sorts of things become possible. That's why, at the first session, I always ask what the patient's dream is, what he or she would love to do, but which is somehow out of reach. Because sometimes I can look back at those early notes and see that the patient has in fact achieved that dream. Then I know that whatever the symptoms, whatever the complaint, acupuncture has achieved its own full potential.

CHAPTER 8

TWO CHALLENGES

At some stage in your first few years you'll face two challenges which are different in kind from any I have mentioned so far, in that they are not to do with the difficulties of diagnosis or treatment, nor even with how you manage your practice, but are about how you react to unusual demands and how you choose to see your role as a practitioner.

The first challenge is when you believe that the Western medical treatment your patient is receiving, or is about to receive, is inappropriate, risky or even damaging to his or her health. Of course, if your patient asks for your advice then it is straightforward – you give it, and if your patient ignores that advice then you carry on treating for as long as you think you can be of help. But what do you do if your advice is not sought? Are you entitled, or obliged, to give it anyway? There is an ethical issue here as well as a professional and practical one, which I can best explain through an example.

I had a patient in his early sixties, a big man, over six feet tall and heavily built. About 20 years ago he had an angioplast and he still has an annual check up both with his doctor and the consultant heart specialist who carried out the procedure. Since then he has been well, busy with work and voluntary projects and playing golf regularly to a good standard. He came to me for acupuncture with a list of minor problems, some back pain, a bout of insomnia, a little heartburn, and he responded well. That was a few years ago. Now he has come complaining that he is terribly tired, can't play more than a few holes of golf before getting exhausted, and is losing interest in the work he used to enjoy.

I ask him what has changed recently and he can't think of anything. Any emotional shocks or struggles? No. Then, feeling slightly guilty that I hadn't kept track of his medication, I ask him if he is taking any medicines. Oh yes. He is taking not one, not two, but three different kinds of drugs for reducing blood pressure, as well as two kinds of statins for cholesterol and an aspirin a day. I was shocked. It sounded an awful lot. So I decided to take his blood pressure.

As I got the equipment ready I reflected on the changes in medical opinion since I qualified. As a student I was taught that the ideal was 140/80 with an increase of ten for every decade over the age of 50. So a norm for him would be about 150/90, maybe a bit more. But recently I had read that nowadays the recommendation was 120/70, with no increase for age. Alright, I thought, there's a bit a leeway here, so somewhere in the region of 140/80 will probably be fine. It was 90/60.

On any criterion, this blood pressure looks too low. Of course, norms and averages must not be taken as truth, for they may not apply to a particular individual. Indeed my father had extraordinarily low blood pressure all his life and was active and dynamic well into his nineties, and there are people who flourish with blood pressure well above what is thought to be healthy. But the point is that my patient was not flourishing. Whether or not it had been a good idea to bring his blood pressure down from its original level, it seemed likely that it had been brought down too far.

'When will you next have it checked by your doctors?' I asked. 'Oh, not for almost a year,' he replied. 'I had a check up only recently.'

Before I go on with the story it is worth pausing to consider the very basic causes of high blood pressure. One is if there is more blood in the arteries than they can comfortably contain; next is if the arteries are too narrow so that the right amount of blood has to pass through too small a tube; and finally if the heart's contraction is so strong that it pushes the blood through the arteries with excessive force. Having set it out like this, it is obvious that a patient will need a different kind of drug depending on which of these is the cause of his high blood pressure. In the first case the usual remedy is a diuretic, a drug which removes fluid from the body, fluid which makes up the blood. If, on the other hand, the arteries have been narrowed by cholesterol then statins are normally prescribed to reduce it. And finally, a class of drugs called beta blockers will ease the power of the heart's contractions.

I supposed it was just possible that my patient had such excessively high blood pressure stemming more or less equally from all three possible causes, that he actually needed all three kinds of medication, but I didn't believe it. I couldn't help thinking that his doctors hadn't bothered to try and isolate the most important cause, and had just decided to give him everything available. What's more, they hadn't even set up any kind of feedback system to be sure that he was being given appropriate dosages. It seemed to me careless at best.

Now, to return to the original question, what should I do about it? He hadn't asked my opinion. He liked and trusted his doctors, indeed one of them was an old friend, and he felt comfortable and secure in their care. Was I to give advice which might upset all that, with consequences I could not foresee? And some patients, though perhaps not him, would feel put in an impossible position, torn between contradictory opinions and with no way of knowing which to believe.

The same basic issue arises with operations. I treated a patient for intermittent back pain while he waited for many months to see a surgeon, who then recommended an operation which would fuse the vertebrae of the spine. 'That'll cure your pain,' the surgeon announced confidently to the patient, who then reported this to me with relief in his voice. What am I to say? That I have seen this operation go wrong and leave people in just as much pain as before but with a serious and incurable loss of mobility? That if my diagnosis is right then the operation won't make any difference because I don't think the pain is caused by compressed discs? That the recovery from the operation is in itself an ordeal and not something to be undertaken lightly? And finally that such drastic intervention can never be reversed so it should only be undertaken if there are really no other options, and I believed there were?

I could multiply the examples, but the point is clear. Is it your job to interfere in your patient's treatment by other practitioners and other forms of medicine?

You will have to find your own responses to these questions. But be aware that they will be asked of you and that they are not easy to answer. Much depends on how you see yourself and how you see your job as an acupuncturist. Are you a doctor, so to speak, or a therapist? Are you an adjunct to your patients' main form of health care or at its centre? As always, and above all, the guiding principle is 'do no harm'. You may not be able to help every one of your patients, nor prevent them from doing things that are not good for them, but you can take care not to cause harm.

For what it is worth, in the first case I did say to my patient that I thought he was being over-medicated and I suggested that he make an appointment with his heart specialist to talk it over. The outcome was a vast reduction in his medication, and he started to be well again almost immediately. In the second case, all I said was that he should think it over carefully because it was a big operation. He had it and it was not a success. It left him with a right leg that was mainly paralysed so he could only walk dragging it along. I often wonder if I should have said more, been more specific, more forceful. What would you have done? And would you be able to rest easy with your decision?

The second challenge concerns some aspect of your character and personality. What happens is that you are confronted by a gap between what you believe in, what you think you are doing as a practitioner or even what sort of person you think you are, and the way you actually behave in the treatment room and treat your patients.

Because we are all different I can't predict the specific content of the challenge you will face but I do know its fundamental shape and basic nature. That's partly because I have been through it myself, and also because I have seen many of the practitioners I have taught having to deal with it too. The bad news is that it can be quite disturbing when you first become aware of it. The good news is that once you've gone through it, then many of the frustrations and irritations you used to experience just don't seem to crop up any more.

Here are a couple of examples to explain what I mean; one from my work before I became an acupuncturist and one since.

I was once in charge of a big project with a staff of about 30 people and a budget of many millions. There was a very important meeting one day with people whose approval was crucial to the project. Unfortunately I was ill that day and could not attend. When I got back to work I asked Ian, a key member of the team and my right hand man, what had happened at the meeting. 'I didn't go,' he said. 'I didn't know what you'd have wanted me to say.' I was astonished. 'But Ian,' I replied. 'You've been with this project since the start. We're all one team. We meet regularly and everyone knows what's happening and where we're going. That's how I set it up and how I've run it.'

Ian smiled. And although it's a very long time ago I can quote his words exactly; 'John,' he said, 'you hold your cards so close to your chest that even you can't see them half the time.'

It was the opposite of what I believed about myself, but as soon as he said it I knew it was true. I trusted his honesty completely and, anyway, his words landed with that unmistakable clunk, which is the sensation of a truth hitting home. There was indeed a gap between what I thought I was like, as a leader, and what I was actually like.

My acupuncture example is very different, but it teaches the same basic lesson. I treated a man in his forties who had quite serious digestive problems; problems which were also a symptom, I thought, of some mental and emotional strain as well. I liked him immediately and looked forward to working with him. After about five treatments he started to be able to eat a much wider range of foods than before, and without the severe cramping pains that he used to have to endure after any meal. That's good, I thought; now we can start to turn our attention to the causes, to the deeper levels and the wider implications of his complaint. For some reason I now forget, we did not make another appointment as usual at the end of the fifth session, maybe I was going away, maybe he didn't have his diary with him. But he never made another appointment and never came back for treatment. I was surprised, disappointed, and even a little hurt. I had thought we were getting on well, that he was enjoying the process and that he was interested in what we were doing together, but it seemed I'd been wrong. Perhaps he really didn't like me and had gone to someone else for treatment.

Time passed and I forgot about it, until some time later when a new patient turned up who had been recommended to me by him. Years later, when this new patient and I knew each other well, I thought it would be alright to ask if she knew why her friend had stopped coming. 'Oh, yes,' she said. 'He felt you'd pushed him away, that you'd made it clear that you'd done all you could for him and didn't want to see him any more.'

It hit me in exactly the same way as Ian's remark. It was shocking to think that I could have been so misunderstood. But at the same time I realised that I must indeed have pushed him away. What on earth was going on?

In a moment I'll explain what was going on, but for now I want to concentrate on this strange phenomenon, that our beliefs about ourselves, about who we are and how we behave, are not necessarily accurate. In fact, I go further. Sooner or later, in some way or other, we find out that they are just plain wrong. We assume that others will always see us as we see ourselves and as we want to be seen, and of course they don't. Sometimes it's because their vision is blurred by whatever is going on for them; but sometimes it's because how we see ourselves is not how we really are.

It is a kind of blind spot. We don't know why what we are doing isn't working, or we simply can't understand why people are reacting to us in the way they do, and because we can't see these things we can't even begin to change them. There's an old saying: If you want to escape from prison, the first thing you must do is to realise that you are in prison, otherwise no escape is possible. Applied here, it means that if there is something about your practice that isn't right, some way in which you don't understand what keeps happening, then the first thing to do is to realise that you are in prison; that there is something about you and how you work which you cannot see. And until you've seen it, it can really make life very difficult.

To go back to my own case, once I'd found out about the patient who felt pushed away I asked around about those patients who had come for a short time and then left, and I found out that many of them had felt the same. What's more, I also discovered that I had quite a few patients who had had the same experience but had kept on coming in spite of it. So what was I doing, and why was I doing it?

Luckily I had a couple of people who were willing to tell me about it. It wasn't that I was uncaring or dismissive. It was a small thing, apparently, but significant. My habit was not to tell my patients how often they needed to come, nor when they should make their next appointment. They took that as an indication that I didn't want to see them again. It's not what I meant, but I could see that it looked like that to them. So why was I doing it? And why did I instinctively not want to change, even when I had found out about it? After some rather uncomfortable self-examination I realised it was because I didn't want anyone to think that I was trying to persuade them to come, trying to get their money off them, trying to get them to be dependent on acupuncture. And that was because I really did want them to like me, to like treatment and to come back for more.

So anxious was I to conceal this neediness that I gave my patients the impression that I didn't want to see them at all!

I have talked to a number of experienced colleagues about this issue, and at one time or another they have all fallen into the same kind of trap, though the specifics were, of course, different. One of them thought she was an absolutely wonderful needler, gentle yet powerful in her technique. What she discovered, after a period when her practice declined sharply, is that many of her patients found her needling too painful to bear, so they stopped coming. It was true that she always hit the point, but only because she often tried two or three times before she got it exactly right, and some of her patients really didn't like being needled repeatedly in almost the same spot. Nor was it true that her needling was gentle. One of her patients was kind enough to describe it like this, 'It feels as if you pick up the point with a crochet hook and then tug it with great difficulty through a hole which is a bit too narrow.'

Another colleague had a spell where he wasn't getting good results at all, and he didn't know why, especially as he took such trouble over his diagnoses. As was normal in his clinic, one of the other practitioners covered for him while he was away on holiday. When he got back he was a bit disturbed to find that his colleague had treated almost all his patients very differently, and was even more concerned to discover that they had all done really well, much better than from any of his recent treatments. Why? Basically because his locum couldn't understand those treatments, based on complex diagnoses, and so had done much simpler work based on the most obvious energy imbalances. The sophisticated diagnoses on which my colleague had prided himself were leading him astray.

These examples point to the main ways of recognising and dealing with this problem. What will trip you up is usually something which you feel is particularly important about you and the way you practise, something of which you are especially proud. Practitioners of five element acupuncture will be very familiar with the idea that your strength is also your weakness, and so it is here. Like the rest of us, you just don't notice things which contradict your view of yourself.

Here are a few ways to spot what you are actually doing as opposed to what you think you are doing.

In most of the stories I have told about this there was a friend or a patient or a colleague who was willing to answer a question honestly, and that is a good way of doing it if you can find someone whose judgement you trust. For some years, a colleague and I used to spend a day every six months or so in each other's treatment rooms, just observing and then giving feedback and sharing ideas about the patients. It was immensely helpful.

Another way of getting a glimpse of what you might be doing is to think back to your clinical teachers and the way they worked. It is easy to pick up their habits, learning to do what they do rather than what they say. One of my teachers used to diagnose not by the methods which he taught us but more by intuition stemming from hands-on work. He would reach a diagnosis, I later realised, without any reference to the theory and he would then make the reasons fit the diagnosis he'd already reached. And without realising what I was doing, I ended up copying him, which was certainly inappropriate for a novice. So think back to your teachers and see if you can pick up the gaps between what they taught you and what you now know constitutes good practice.

Finally, you can try jotting down a few sentences about your work, starting each with a phrase like, 'I think it is really important to...' or, 'In my practice I always...' or, 'I believe my strong point as a practitioner is...' and then write down the opposite of each of these. What I have in mind is repeating the sentence but starting with, 'I think it is really important but I usually don't...' or, 'In my practice I believe I always do the following, but actually...' or, 'I suspect that my weak point as a practitioner is...' and seeing if you get that clunk, that sinking feeling of a truth revealed. If you are brave enough you could even try showing those opposites to a trusted colleague or patient, and see how they respond.

Once you've spotted the gap then you have the opportunity to change, to make what you do consistent with what you believe you should be doing. But it is worth noticing that there is another option. You can instead change what you believe in order to bring it in line with what you actually do. If it is the gap which is the problem, then it can be narrowed from either end.

Take the example of the way I pushed my patients away. At the time, when I spotted this behaviour, I made great efforts to change it. It didn't occur to me then, as it does now, that I could also have decided that, actually, I did want to push my patients away. I could have said to myself that the truth was I obviously didn't much like having patients year in year out, that it seemed that as soon as they showed real signs of improvement I lost interest. So perhaps it would be better to be upfront about it. I could have decided that in future I would say to them, 'I'm happy to treat you for a while, but there will come a point when I think I'll have done all I can for you, and I'll want to stop treating – then I'll recommend someone else if you want.'

Nothing wrong with that, if that's how I wanted to work. The problem only arose when I try to run my practice according to some belief which turned out not to be true. It was when I was unclear, when I gave unintentional or contradictory messages, that everyone got confused and disappointed.

It may sound as if this is just a lazy way of dealing with the problem, one that means you don't have to change, but there may be real wisdom in choosing this option. It may be that you are hampered, not helped, by a sense of duty or obligation or commitment to some style of practice which doesn't actually suit you, and that this is undermining your work. Perhaps what you actually do is better, or at least just as good as what you think you should do. A well-known gardener once gave this advice to people creating a new garden, 'Don't put down any paths in the first year. Wait and see where people walk and then lay out the paths where they've actually walked.' It's the same idea.

Reading this now you may wonder why I have placed such emphasis on this issue. It may seem to be just another part of the life-long learning that you know this practice to be. But it is qualitatively different from discovering that your pulse-taking skills need to improve, or that you don't really understand Internal Wind, or even that you need to learn a whole new diagnostic system. What is so hard about this challenge is that when you face it you are brought up against some aspect of yourself which you normally do not notice and which you do not care to recognise even when it is plain to see. It can be very uncomfortable. And because it involves personal rather than professional issues, your training may not have prepared you for it, nor taught you how to manage it. So dealing with it can be difficult.

As ever, though, forewarned is forearmed. It will help a lot that when you are confronted in this way you will know that it is normal, that you are not inadequate nor unsuited to the work, and that most practitioners before you have had to cope with it too.

When this arises for you, it is awfully tempting to take a quick peek at the issue but never to confront it fully, which pretty much guarantees that it will dog you for years. Much better, I think, to tackle it head on, as soon as possible, and with a commitment to resolving it. Remember too that with all these kinds of self-examination, the reality is never as bad as the fantasy. It's like the skeleton in the cupboard; much less frightening once the door is open. So do whatever you have to do to summon up your courage, but know that your worst fears will not be realised.

And finally, have faith that there are large rewards awaiting you when you have done it. You will find that your work will move to a whole new level, free of a constraint which, without you knowing it, has held you back for a long time. And held you back not merely from you at your best as an acupuncturist, but as a person too.

CHAPTER 9

THE NEXT STAGE

So far I have been describing some of the steps you will need to take as you follow the path from anxious novice to confident practitioner. I remember vividly the time I realised that it had happened to me. It was a Monday, I had worked through a full day, I was walking home, and I suddenly noticed that something had changed, that this evening was not like all the other evenings I had walked back from the clinic. The difference was that for the first time ever I was not worrying about a single one of the treatments I had done that day. Previously I had always had doubts, had always spent the journey wondering if a diagnosis was right, if I should have used moxa on someone, feeling foolish that I hadn't thought of a point which now seemed obviously right for a particular patient, and so on. All the way to my front door. But on that Monday evening – nothing. And the phrase came to me, I know what I'm doing now.

This will happen to you too. Indeed, the point of this book is to help you to get to this stage a little more quickly and a little more smoothly than I did. What I didn't think to ask myself, as I strolled home, was, 'What next?' I wish I had, because it would have helped me to be aware of what might be in store for me and it would have helped me to take the next steps as an acupuncturist. So in this last chapter I want to look ahead, to give you some indication of the choices you have before you, and the demands that will be made of you, if you want to go deeper in your practice.

In the years before I became competent I had the good fortune to meet three truly great practitioners, genuine masters of this form of medicine. I was privileged to have long discussions with one of them, to observe another at work and to be treated by the third. I learned so much from them without even realising it. For example, one of them took pulses much more often and for much longer than I had been taught, and instinctively I found myself copying her. Another of them worked so simply it was a revelation. He once treated me by tonifying LI 11 on the right, and nothing else. This treatment made absolutely no sense at all according to any of the theories I had learned, and yet I felt wonderful afterwards. Gradually I had the sense to ask myself, 'What do these great practitioners know that I don't?'

The answer to that question turned out to be extremely useful. In describing what I learned from them, I don't intend to suggest that you need to copy them. It's more that some of the features of the way they work will stimulate your interest and excitement, and others will not; and that will be a good guide for you in the future. Over the years there will be many opportunities for continuing professional development and you won't be able to take them all, so it will be useful to have some idea of the direction you want to go in as a practitioner and some pointers to the way in which you want to excel.

First, I noticed that they collected more information from their patients than I did, and more useful information too. It wasn't that they spent longer talking to them, nor even that their questions were obviously more penetrating and perceptive than mine. It was that all three of them listened better than I did. It was common for them to be quiet for long periods, just nudging the patient to carry on when he or she stopped talking. They noticed what the patients didn't say as well as what they did; noticed when the words and the emotion with which they were spoken, even the tone of voice that was used, were incongruous; they registered changes in posture, such as looking away, and linked them to what the patient was saying at the time. They even noticed different kinds of silence, seeing a real distinction between a patient who regularly looked down when he fell quiet and one whose eyes turned upwards. It made me realise that I needed to learn to listen, because I wanted to be able to hear what I was being told behind and beyond the words that my patient can find. There is a lovely sentence which sums this up perfectly: 'My mother...understood... that the declared meaning of a spoken sentence is only its overcoat, and the real meaning lies beneath its scarves and buttons' (Carey 1988, pp.189–190).

It is a skill, one which few people know how to do instinctively, but it can be learned and it has some surprising effects.

To explain how this works, there is really no substitute for trying it. You can start with a friend or colleague. Sit opposite each other. You each decide on a topic you want to talk about, which should be something important to you, even something which puzzles or worries you. One of you then talks about that topic for five minutes (experience has shown that is a good length of time) and the other just listens.

When I say, just listens, I mean that there are to be no interruptions at all. That means no questions or comments, nor any gestures like smiling, sighing or shrugging. That's because these all communicate what the listener is thinking, and that is a distraction for the speaker. We all tend to alter what we say to please the person we are talking to, for example by swerving away from a subject if we get the message that it is boring, and so on. The point is that the speaker must be allowed to say what he or she really wants to say, needs to say, without being influenced to alter it in order to please the listener. Therefore the listener also needs to keep eye contact with the speaker (for as long as the speaker chooses to look at the listener), because if the listener looks away and stares at the floor or the ceiling, that conveys the unmistakable message that he or she is bored or is thinking of something else, which again will influence the speaker.

Up to this point, the exercise shows how the act of really listening alters what people feel able to say, encouraging them to reveal more than they usually do. This is the real secret of how the masters find out so much about their patients so quickly. And something else, something rather remarkable, often happens too. Freed from the need to be interesting or pleasing, the speaker finds him- or herself saying things that come as quite a surprise. 'I didn't know I thought that until I said it,' people often comment after this exercise, 'but once I did, I knew it was true.' It is, in short, a way for a patient to learn more about him- or herself, what he or she really wants or needs, and that can be an extremely powerful part of the healing process.

The next stage of the exercise comes at the end of the five minutes, when the listener has to sum up what the speaker has said. Then the speaker says whether or not the listener has left anything out, made any mistakes, and most important of all, whether the summary captures the real meaning of what was said. If not (and it is rare for any beginner to get it right first time) then the listener tries again until the speaker is satisfied that he or she has been heard. It can be almost embarrassing, but it is certainly revealing, to discover how often what we hear is not what the speaker was trying to tell us. This is basically because, as soon as words are spoken, we interpret them to fit in with what we think and believe, which may not be at all what the speaker thinks and believes.

And here is another lesson taught by the great practitioners. Their patients feel heard. They feel that someone has understood them and knows what they are going through. They do not feel that they have been ignored, patronised, categorised, bullied or made to feel inadequate (all reports from my patients about how they have experienced some medical interviews). And being properly heard is in itself a very powerful aid to healing, because being ill is a lonely business. Family and friends can be wonderfully helpful and supportive, but most patients don't want to burden them with their complaints, especially if they are chronic ones. Listening properly tells the patient that he or she is not alone.

The master practitioners also gathered an enormous amount of information through touch. It isn't easy to describe in words how they do this, but the essence of it was that I saw how they would adjust their touch until it was comfortable for the patient. More than comfortable actually, for the touch itself became part of the healing. So the masters were doing two things at once. By finding out exactly how each patient liked to be touched they were finding out a great deal about the state of his or her energy. I once saw one of them handling a big strong young man, a rugby player, as if he were a fragile old lady. After the treatment I asked him why he had done that. He smiled, 'I was deceived at first,' he said, 'but that young man's energy body is so delicate I almost felt I had to hold my breath as I touched it.' I'm not sure anyone could have discovered this except by finding out how he liked to be touched. With another patient, a dynamic business woman, his touch was very firm but also very deliberate and slow. 'She is always rushing ahead,' he commented afterwards, 'it's part of her lifestyle and she's become accustomed to it. But it isn't really who she is, and it doesn't really suit her.' And I had indeed noticed that this patient had relaxed unusually deeply during the treatment; perhaps she came for that as much as for anything the needles could do for her.

You can learn a lot about touch by being alert to your patient's response to what you do. If you mark out back shu points with your patient sitting on the couch, for example, does he lean in to your touch or away from it? When you pick up your patient's hand to take her pulses, does she hold it herself or is she willing to let go and let you take the weight of it? And if she does keep hold of it, can you adjust your touch so she feels able to relax?

Another direction in which you may choose to develop your skills is in working with what is often called psychosomatic illness. As it is such an important phenomenon, and so common, I want to say a little about it before I turn to how the masters manage it.

The starting place is a quotation from one of America's foremost cancer surgeons, not someone who can be accused of a lack of knowledge or understanding of scientific medicine, nor of lack of respect for the achievements of the operating theatre. He says, 'Years of experience have taught me that cancer and indeed nearly all diseases are psychosomatic. This may sound strange to people accustomed to thinking that psychosomatic ailments are not truly "real" but, believe me, they are' (Siegel 1988, p.111).

To say that an illness is psychosomatic doesn't mean that the patient's physical symptoms are all in the mind; they are usually and most definitely in the body too. Nor does it mean that the illness can only be cured or alleviated through psychological change, for in my experience you can relieve profoundly psychosomatic illness by altering the energy state which is keeping that illness locked in place.

What it does mean is that making sense of an illness can be a way of dissolving its mystery, answering the questions we all ask when we are ill: 'Why?' 'Why me?' 'Why should I be so afflicted?' All the masters helped their patients to come to some kind of understanding of their condition, which in itself can bring about deep and lasting change.

Here are a few examples. I tell them briefly and simply, though, as you can imagine, it can take a long time, through many treatments, to get to this clarity.

A woman develops a curious skin condition, not quite like any in the books. It turns out to be an allergic reaction to particular foods, all of which she used to be able to eat without any trouble. After talking in detail about what each of these foods might mean to her, her history with them so to speak, she suddenly realises that they constituted the meal she was eating when her husband told her he was having an affair. No wonder they have become poisonous to her, for she took them in at the same time as she absorbed something that harmed her.

A man struggles with depression. He often feels weighed down. The father he adored, the father who died ten years ago, left a substantial fortune to his second wife and his stepson and practically nothing to his only son. His son denies that he is angry or resentful about this; nothing, it seems, can diminish the devotion he feels towards his father's memory. After many months of treatment the practitioner learns that he sleeps on the top floor of his house, directly under the attic where he has stored all his father's papers, the will, the details of the estate, old letters and so on. It is not hard to imagine that this might not be good for him; that he might feel lighter, physically and emotionally, if he threw the papers away, or at least moved them to the basement instead.

An air stewardess in her mid thirties comes for treatment because she suffers from bloating in the lower burner, periods that go on for a week, and occasional incontinence. She has been to her doctor and had all sorts of tests but none of them showed anything abnormal. At first she was pleased with this outcome, glad to know that there was nothing wrong, but as the symptoms gradually got worse she became more and more worried. To her acupuncturist, all the symptoms pointed to a weakness in the functioning of her Spleen. Treatment was effective at first, and for short periods, but her symptoms kept returning. Probing a little more deeply, she said that she had been brought up on a farm and had loved it, and that she relaxed by growing vegetables in her garden. Perhaps her Earth element was rebelling against leaving the ground continually, and the only real, long-term remedy for her, would be to give up her job.

What all three examples have in common is that it can be difficult to find out about these crucial aspects of the patient's condition. It is quite hard to imagine how the normal conversation between patient and practitioner could have got around to the fact that the patient was sleeping directly underneath the papers of a father who had disparaged and belittled him. Or, to take another example, in my own treatment one day I commented that at a meal with one of my daughters I had taken my jacket off and then put it on again, and repeated the process quite a few times. My practitioner pounced on that seemingly innocuous comment, and a few minutes later I knew something important about my relationship with that daughter and about my propensity for catching colds.

The first lesson, once again, is to learn to listen.

The other thing that these stories have in common is that treatment will only really work once the patient has understood something about his or her life. It can be at the relatively simple level of explaining the function of the Liver in Chinese medicine, and hence why a patient always gets a migraine when he's had alcohol, coffee and chocolate the night before. Because we are so used to the functions of the organs and the location of the meridians, it is easy to underestimate what a revelation this kind of explanation can be, and how profoundly it can affect a patient's life. For it can offer a way out of what seemed an inescapable affliction. But sometimes, as in the examples above, guidance at a deeper level is needed.

There are two parts to this. The first is understanding the mental, emotional or spiritual aspect of the patient's illness, such as the connection between the skin complaint and the traumatic meal. And the second is finding a way of helping the patient to collaborate in the process of change.

You will treat people who believe that illness comes from outside and hits them for no reason at all, so they will not accept any suggestion of psychosomatic cause. You will treat people who are defensive, feeling that your attempt to explain what has happened to them is intrusive and unwarranted. You will treat people who know perfectly well, once you have told them, that their condition needs to be treated every two weeks or so, but they still only come every couple of months. I could give many more examples; the point is that it takes real care, much thought, and a great deal of skill to find a way to help patients like these. It is absolutely no good lecturing them, nor will it help if you get frustrated with them. The trick is to see their inability or unwillingness to help themselves as part of the energetic pattern which is keeping them stuck in their illness; and if you can do that, then you can treat that pattern. This, I think, is what the master practitioners do. They focus on removing the stuckness in order to liberate the patient's own healing power.

This leads me to describe a fundamental quality shared by the three practitioners I watched. In my early years in practice I noticed that I worked well with a certain quite narrow group of people; those, I suppose, who were more or less like me and who shared similar attitudes and values. But others I found hard. I didn't really make contact with them or appreciate them, and they tended to have a treatment or two, but then didn't come back. By contrast, as I watched the masters at work, sometimes with people who were being grudging, recalcitrant or even quite hostile, they managed to create a real bond with every single one of them. And then I saw those same, difficult patients slowly begin to ease their rigidity, saw them respond to their practitioner and relax into the process of treatment and of healing.

It's a matter, I think, of how the practitioners regarded their patients. In talking to me about their patients they didn't judge or criticise. They didn't say things like, 'She really does go on and on...' or, 'He is so needy that he always...' or, 'What does he expect? He's bound to have a headache if he drinks that much...' or, 'I gave her a treatment for her shoulder and the silly woman went out and played tennis straight afterwards...' Instead they demonstrated, over and over again, a profound acceptance of their patients, just as they were, with all their failings and foolishnesses, all their defences and their neuroses. They were living examples of the following teaching: 'If the doctor wishes to help a human being he must accept him as he is. And he can do this in reality only when he has already seen and accepted himself as he is. Perhaps this sounds simple, but simple things are always the most difficult' (Jung 1989, p.271).

We all find some patients hard to accept as they are. If Jung is right, these patients will be the ones who, somehow or other, alert us to an aspect of our own nature of which we are unaware, and which we are reluctant or unwilling to see. Reacting to them is really a reaction to ourselves, to our own hidden natures. To learn to do good work with whoever walks into your treatment room does require a level of personal development and a willingness to face your assumptions and prejudices, which will serve you well not only as a practitioner but as a person.

In the end, what this all amounts to is that the great practitioners always work holistically. They don't separate their patient's minds from their bodies, their spirits from their emotions, their illnesses from their health, nor indeed do they separate themselves from their patients. They see it all as part of trying to deal with the pain, illness and disability inherent in a human life. Nor indeed do they make distinctions in the treatment room between what they are trying to achieve with needles or with talking, with touch or with silence. It is all in service to bringing about a change in the patient's energy.

And because they see it this way, they are modest. Of course, they know they are highly skilled and experienced but they don't think of themselves as healers and they don't think it is they who heal. They would heartily agree with Albert Schweitzer, possibly the most famous and revered doctor of the twentieth century.

> When I asked Dr Schweitzer how he accounted for the fact that anyone could possibly expect to become well after having been treated by a witch doctor, he said I was asking him to divulge a secret that doctors have carried around with them ever since Hippocrates. 'But I'll tell you anyway,' he said, his face still illuminated by that half smile. 'The witch doctor succeeds for the same reason all the rest of us succeed. Each patient carries his own doctor inside him. They come to us not knowing that truth. We are at our best when we give the doctor who resides within each patient a chance to go to work. (Cousins 1981, pp.68–69)

CONCLUSION

How do you talk about your patients, even to yourself? Do you ever think, for example, that you are treating your patient's asthma, or hypertension or irritable bowel? Do you say to yourself, this patient has Liver Qi stagnation? I believe it is a mistake to think you are treating a patient's asthma or hypertension, even to think that your patient has Liver Qi stagnation.

Imagine someone comes to you because he has a number of symptoms commonly associated with hypertension, and his doctor has told him that he needs to bring his blood pressure down. Before going on to take the prescribed medication, he has decided to see if acupuncture can help. You find out about him and his lifestyle, you ask about the symptoms, you take his pulses and look at his tongue. You come to the conclusion that there are signs of Liver Yang rising but the fundamental cause of his condition is probably Kidney Yin deficiency. Now, when you formulate your treatment plan what do you think you are treating, the hypertension or the Kidney Yin deficiency?

If it is the first, then I think you may lose your focus. You will naturally pay more attention to the numbers on his blood pressure monitor than to any change in his energetic state. Your criteria of success will be whether or not his blood pressure comes down, rather than whether treatment has re-established the right balance between Kidney Yin and Kidney Yang, and whether that calms the Liver Yang rising. Also, by treating his blood pressure as if it were separable from his overall health and well-being, you will have lost sight of the fundamentally holistic nature of acupuncture. Treating his blood pressure, indeed treating any specific condition defined in Western medical terms, will lead you astray.

Here is a different example but it relates to the same basic issue. Do you say to yourself, 'This patient has Liver Qi stagnation (or any of the other syndromes)?' If so, then you are effectively equating these syndromes with a disease; saying that a patient has Kidney Yin deficiency, for example, in the same way as you might say he has rheumatoid arthritis, or diabetes or cancer. I suggest that this too will lead you astray. The acupuncturist's way of looking at it is different. It is to see what we call Liver Qi stagnation as an energetic response, one way among many in which people react to the pressures and stresses of life.

Every patient responds to these pressures in a particular way. To some extent, that response might be thought of as constitutional, as an energetic disposition with which he or she was born (or which was acquired very early in life). To some extent the response might be a learned behaviour, something that once seemed to be an effective survival strategy in order to get through some crisis or trauma, but which has now become as unhelpful as it is habitual.

The point is that if you think your patient *has* Liver Qi stagnation then your approach will be to try to take it away and generally act upon it as if it is a medical dysfunction, to be cured or alleviated by outside intervention. If on the other hand you see his Liver Qi stagnation as a learned response to life's difficulties then there are some important consequences.

One is that you won't believe that you can take it away with your treatments, for under the appropriate conditions it is likely to re-emerge. The second is that although you can certainly help, only the patient can change this response. And finally, it follows that treatment then becomes a collaboration between the two of you to identify the causes, the possible alternative responses, and the points which can best help him change. Essentially, what you will be doing is identifying a particular route back to health and, with your needles, discovering and then prodding him or her along the path that leads there.

These consequences derive from a coherent and consistent view of the body, one which speaks of the nature of its ailments and the nature of health. Like all such views it is both partial and revealing. To a chemist, for example, the body is an exquisitely complex chemical factory, producing enzymes and proteins, hormones and haemoglobin; a view which shows him how to synthesise drugs which can help the body to heal. The equivalent perspective for an acupuncturist, in short, is that the body is a field of forces, identical to those which govern all living matter and which work together in a balanced way. Illness, therefore, is a state of imbalance, and the job of the practitioner is to restore balance.

It is so vital not to lose sight of the fact that all our work stems from this core perspective. I am not saying that we are always able to restore balance, nor that it is always possible even in principle to do so. There are some energy states which are so far out of balance that they cannot be brought back again; which is simply to say that there are some illnesses and diseases which are immune to acupuncture treatment. But if we abandon the core of our work in an attempt to copy the attitudes, the styles and the methodologies of Western medicine then we will no longer be doing the best we can for our patients.

In the face of a patient with a really clear Western diagnosis like a stomach ulcer or labyrinthitis or hepatitis, it is sometimes hard to keep faith with our method and look for imbalances in the patient's energy rather than think of specific points for the stomach, the ear or the liver. Especially when we've tried treating the imbalance and it did not help. But it is simply the case that your treatments, like any other kind of medical treatments, will not always work. That is no reason to give up on them, no reason to abandon your belief in what you are doing, and absolutely no reason to shift to the illusory safety of using needles in a way that is not based on the accumulated wisdom of thousands of years of skilled clinical experience.

Have faith, and trust in energy. It's real, it's wonderful and it works.

REFERENCES

Beinfield, H. and Korngold, E. (1991) *Between Heaven and Earth: A Guide to Chinese Medicine.* New York, NY, Ballentine Books.

Carey, P. (1988) *Oscar and Lucinda.* London: Faber and Faber.

Cousins, N. (1981) *Anatomy of an Illness.* New York, NY, Bantam Books. First published 1979.

Darby, M. (2003) 'Professor J. R. Worsley. A personal tribute.' *European Journal of Oriental Medicine 4,* 3, 34.

Dass, R. and Gorman, P. (1992) *How Can I Help?* London: Rider. First published 1985.

Hunt, V. V. (1989) *Infinite Mind: Science of the Human Vibrations of Consciousness.* Malibu, CA, Malibu Publishing.

Jung, C. G. (1989) *Modern Man in Search of a Soul.* London: Ark Paperbacks. First published 1933.

Ramen, R. N. (1989) 'The Search for Healing.' In R. Carlson and B. Shield (eds) *Healers on Healing.* Los Angeles, CA, Jeremy P. Tarcher.

Siegel, B. S. (1988) *Love, Medicine and Miracles.* London: Arrow. First published 1986.